HOW TO COPE
SUCCESSFULLY WITH

MENOPAUSE

DR JOAN MCCLELLAND

Wellhouse Publishing Ltd

First published in Great Britain in 2001 by
Wellhouse Publishing Ltd
31 Middle Bourne Lane
Lower Bourne
Farnham
Surrey GU10 3NH

Reprinted in 2003, 2004. Revised 2006

DISCLAIMER

The aim of this book is to provide general information only and should
not be treated as a substitute for the medical advice of your doctor or
any other health care professional. The publisher and author is not
responsible or liable for any diagnosis made by a reader based on the
contents of this book. Always consult your doctor if you are in any way
concerned about your health.

A catalogue record for this book is available from the British Library

ISBN 1 903784 05 0

Printed and bound in Great Britain by
Creative Design & Print, Wales

Introduction

The menopause is an event to welcome - the opening of a gateway into a fresh, new, stimulating chapter in your life. At last you can be your own person, uncluttered by what used to be called 'the curse' - the monthly physical and emotional disturbance that always seemed to come at the wrong time. You can say goodbye to PMT, water retention, period pain and a host of psychological symptoms - irritability, depression and chronic tension. You will no longer be at risk of becoming anaemic from the monthly loss of blood.

Nor are you, at this stage, caught up in the frenetic drive to compete for men and jobs that bugged you at 30, the niggling worry about contraceptive failure, nor the balancing act between family and career. Your children still need you, but more often now as a wise counsellor than a workhorse.

This exciting stage in your personal development comes plumb in the middle of the most productive period of adult life, the two decades from 40 to 60 - currently the peak age for the menopause in the UK is 50 years and 9 months. Three-quarters of scientific advances are made by 50 to 60-year-olds, while novelists' output is running at a high, and career women, like men, are reaching their highest earning capacity. It is a time of opportunity or for consolidation - whichever attracts you.

The menopause is a vantage point from which to take stock, reviewing your earlier life and learning its lessons, and looking ahead to any heights you want to scale, or the quieter achievement of new interests and the deepening of your relationships. There is plenty of time - 30 or 40 years, minimum - to fit in all you want. On the personal front, which as a woman is always with you, whatever your other work and responsibilities, you are at a crucial stage. Among the items you may have to cope with are:

1. Teenaged and newly adult children in serious need of guidance and support - whatever they might say!
2. Marriage: the fabric has often become dangerously threadbare at this juncture, and running repairs are urgently needed - or a divorce achieved without bloodletting.
3. Your sex life may be at crisis point, too, having become no more riveting than cleaning your teeth. It will need a fresh infusion of magic.
4. Your own parents are beginning to act their age, and the balance of power, or at least of responsibility, is shifting from their shoulders to yours. You will find them looking to you for help and advice - for instance with the intricacies of the Internet.
5. You may have been turned, willy-nilly, into a grandmother, perhaps with hands-on involvement, producing a conflict over your job and your inclinations.

It would be impossible to cope successfully with all of this, plus have some

fun and satisfaction for yourself, if it were not for the menopause. This time to off-load inessentials, like your periods. For your partner as w yourself, this is the time to rejig your lifestyle, for long-term health and ciency. Enlarge the slots for exercise and, especially, rearrange your d is deadly to your figure, your joints and your arteries to continue wit food intake you needed at 20 and 30.

Don't be misled by the downbeat pronouncements of the pessin many of them men, who write off the menopause as made up of dec deterioration and loss. Our grandmothers' phrase, 'the change of li more accurate, since the essence is change not loss. The only thing have lost is the ability to have babies - and hopefully you will have don already, if you wanted to. It is only in the West that the menopause has tive connotations. In much of Asia and Africa it is seen as an achieve and boon. In sub-Saharan Africa and Ethiopia women greatly increa status when they pass the change, while in Rajasthan they are rele from purdah and may mix freely with the opposite sex for the first They are considered wise enough now to give guidance to younger pe

Men, who age faster than women, make a big thing of celebrating half-century. This is not the way of women. We are far too wise to be strained by dates and ages. If we want to stop counting at 49 - why Better still to ignore the crude and meaningless numbers and live a feel. Middle age is a state of mind - don't fall into it.

Meanwhile your body is making some sensible adjustments to fit its your new life, and while this is happening you may get some tire symptoms. Not everyone is affected, but if you are among the un 80%, you have the consolation of knowing that this stage is tempora one is menopausal at 90! Besides, if your enjoyment of life is impaired, there is HRT - hormone replacement therapy - to rescue a range of other treatments if that does not suit you.

You are entering an important and fascinating phase in your life, di from anything you have experienced before. To get the very best out c need to work in harmony with what nature is trying to do, and for t need to understand your own body. Together, in this book, let us e the interesting and useful facts about your body and how it functic adapts to your needs. Your feelings, too, need special understanding turning point in your life.

Recent research has shown a new use for oestrogen patches, the proved useful in some cases for treating men with advanced canc prostate. These patches have shown a lower risk of side effects t tablets previously prescribed. Women too may have side effects v trogen, the implication of the male studies is that women may als from these patches. Trials are currently under way.

Chapter 1

What Is the Menopause and Why Is It So Important?

The menopause is a revolution that affects your body, your mind and your emotions – a major milestone in the great journey of life through birth, puberty, motherhood, menopause, maturity and what are known as the third and fourth ages.

To be precise, it is the date of your last period. You will not recognize it when it happens, since you have to let a year pass without periods to know that this was the last one. A century ago the most common age for the menopause was two or three years earlier than it is today. Now the peak age for the last period is 50 years and 9 months, but anywhere between your early 40s and your mid-50s is within the normal range.

A premature menopause is one that occurs before the age of 40. This is a trait that often runs in families, and it is important to be aware of it because it is associated with an increased risk of osteoporosis and coronary heart disease.

An artificial menopause is one that can be produced at any time, for instance if the ovaries are removed for medical reasons (*oophorectomy*), or the egg-cells are destroyed incidentally by radiotherapy or chemotherapy. If you have had mumps involving the ovaries, that also harms the egg-cells and brings the menopause forwards.

Smokers lose their egg-cells faster than other people, and their menopause comes about two years sooner than average. This also happens with those who have had a hysterectomy in which the ovaries were left undisturbed.

The Perimenopause

This includes a period of two or three years running up to the menopause and also the few years following – *peri-* is Greek for 'surrounding'. Another term is the *climacteric*, meaning a ladder leading up to a climax. During the first part the ovaries are gradually running out of egg-cells, and as a result are producing less oestrogen. This may result in light, infrequent or irregular periods – commonly the first indication of the approaching change. There may be other symptoms, too, also caused by the fluctuating levels of oestrogen in your blood. For instance there may be flooding one

Contents

	Introduction	4
1.	What Is the Menopause and Why Is It So Important?	6
2.	Know Your Way Around	10
3.	How the System Works: The Controls	13
4.	Symptoms and Signs: Local	16
5.	Symptoms and Signs: General	24
6.	Psychological and Emotional Effects	27
7.	Osteoporosis	36
8.	Heart and Artery Disease	44
9.	Hormone Replacement Therapy: Why Should You Take It?	51
10.	Hormone Replacement Therapy: How to Take It	58
11.	Hormone Replacement Therapy: Side-effects	69
12.	Exercise as Treatment	79
13.	Treatment Other than HRT	85
14.	Alternative Therapies	94
15.	Herbal Medicines	101
16.	Sex and the Menopause	106
17.	Contraception	113
18.	Eating for Health in the Change	119
	Useful Addresses	126
	Index	127

month and no bleeding at all the next, and general effects such as headaches and insomnia.

After the actual menopause there is inevitably a period of adjustment, including the revving-up of oestrogen production from the adrenal glands and fatty tissue, compensating in part for the fall-off from the ovaries. There are also significant changes in your breasts, womb, muscles, bones and mind. Strictly speaking, this is all part of the perimenopause, but usually when we use the term 'menopause' we are referring to the whole period of building up to the menopause and the immediate consequences.

What Makes the Menopause So Important?

The menopause is a watershed between two major phases in your life. The first half covered growing up, education, perhaps finding a partner and perhaps bringing up children. During all of this, other people may have called the shots – your parents, your teacher, your partner and your own family. In the second part, your new life is, for the first time, in your hands.

The change involves a complete shake-up of roles – within the family, socially and at work:

● At home you are no longer just 'Mum'.
● Socially you are not now one of those women whose favourite topic of conversation is their children and who are always having to dash off and collect them from school or a party, and whose holidays are geared to what the youngest can do.
● Work-wise you are now able to branch out, chase up what interests you and take your career seriously.

New Priorities

This is the time when you need a brand-new set of health priorities, which are nothing to do with the monthly rhythm, and call for big changes in your lifestyle and diet. The watchword is PREVENTION. It is not that you have an illness, but this is the time to take sensible precautions against developing those baddies that could spoil your life in your 60s, 70s and 80s.

Osteoporosis and coronary heart/artery problems are the two big risks that loom up as you enter the menopausal stage, and there are other pitfalls you must be aware of and sidestep.

Preparing for the Menopause

It is amazing that there is so little advice on offer about preparing for something as momentous as the menopause. The way you plan your lifestyle now will have repercussions for the next 30 or 40 years, and in the short term can help you to avoid or diminish the menopausal symptoms themselves.

When should you start? Ideally this would be in your early 40s, since by 40 your ovaries will already have begun, secretly, to adjust to the time when you are not planning to have more babies. Your body will give you a reminder that something strange is happening, with extra heavy or short, light periods, haywire timing or subtle changes in your mood.

This is the time to ditch bad habits once and for all, before they do any serious harm:

- Smoking is the worst, directly responsible for cancers of the lung and larynx, and contributing to several others, including those affecting women in particular: breast, ovary and, also womb and colon cancer. Colds that 'go to your chest' and a smoker's cough are urgent signals of danger ahead.

- Overweight. This is the age and stage for the dreaded middle-aged spread to take hold. If you do not deal with it before your menopause is established, you will find it much more difficult to shift the unwanted fat – especially in the typically female sites: hips, thighs and your tummy below the waist. It is a matter of more exercise and better chosen food – with the emphasis on fruit and vegetables and a cutback on fats, the sweet and sugary, and most convenience and junk foods. However, there are benefits from being slightly plump – you are at less risk of osteoporosis and your skin is likely to retain its underlay of colloid and look blooming.

- Constipation. This often becomes a problem around the time of the menopause. It makes any abdominal discomfort worse and leads to headaches and general sluggishness. It is important to adjust your diet and the amount of exercise you take so that your bowels act regularly, with only the occasional reminder, before you go into the menopausal phase – when everything runs to a slower rhythm. The Victorians advised taking the mildly laxative herb aloe vera for menopausal women. This is available today in health-food stores. On the diet front, you will need more fibre – fruit and vegetables again, plus bran, whole-grain cereals, oats and wholemeal bread, with plenty to drink.

There are also specific disorders which some sensible adjustments to your diet and lifestyle can help you to avoid:

Osteoporosis
After your menopause you are likely to be offered hormone replacement therapy, HRT, to replace some of the oestrogen that is lacking. In advance

preparation for the change, there are two helpful ploys to keep your bones strong and healthy:

- Calcium, as found in dairy products, plus dietary supplements of vitamin D (in fish liver oils)
- Weight-bearing exercise, such as walking, golf and tennis

Heart and Artery Disease
This includes coronary heart attack, high blood pressure and the danger of a stroke. Being overweight and smoking increase the risks, but on the positive side a diet based on fruit and vegetables, with plenty of antioxidants (contained in green, yellow and red vegetables) reduces the risks. Supplements of vitamin E also help, while oatmeal is officially recommended by Government advisers. Saturated animal fats make matters worse by clogging the arteries. Now is the time to change to one of the wide choice of polyunsaturate spreads.

Problems in the Uterus
Now that it has lost its top job (housing a foetus), other conditions tend to crop up in the womb, for instance fibroids, which are non-cancerous tumours in the muscle, and endometriosis, a disorder of the womb lining. Much less often a cancer may develop, so it is very important to tell your doctor if you have any bleeding that you are not sure is due to a period.

Psychological and Emotional Difficulties
The menopause is notorious as a time when women can become moody and irritable, or downright depressed. Dr Quain, in 1885, advised that women in the climacteric should be shielded from any 'excitement'. Today we would call it stress. It is certainly wise to avoid stress when your body and mind are likely to be in a certain amount of turmoil. This is not the moment to move house, swap jobs or go in for divorce. You are likely to have enough of the unavoidable pressures – with children leaving home, your parents suddenly becoming old and perhaps developing serious illnesses, and your own natural anxiety about the menopause.

The main stress-busters are confiding relationships – so nurture your friendships and, where necessary, repair and strengthen communications with your partner and children. If you do not already have a job outside the home, this is a good time to begin – voluntary work if you prefer. It gives you a different focus now that the family does not absorb so much of your mind.

When you have prepared for it by planning and establishing a healthy, interesting and fulfilling lifestyle in advance, you can meet the menopause with confidence.

Chapter 2

Know Your Way Around

The genital system is the source of desire, sex, pleasure and babies. Each part of it has a role to play.

External Arrangements

These, collectively, are known as the *vulva* (Latin for the cover of a seed) and, unlike the situation in men, they are hidden. From the back you see only a woman's buttocks, and from the front all that is visible is the *mons pubis*, where the pubic bones meet in the midline, covered by a pad of fibrous tissue and the pubic hair. This is coarse and curly, and stops in a straight line across the lower edge of the abdomen. It is special – children do not have it before they reach puberty, and older people gradually lose it. It depends on a good supply of sex hormones, oestrogen in particular.

The Labia
Between your legs are two folds of skin with a lining of fat, the *labia majora*, which feel to the touch like ordinary skin. *Labia* is Latin for lips, and *majora* means that the labia majora are bigger than the *labia minora*. These are thin folds of delicate, pink skin which lie within the *labia majora*. They are very sensitive compared with the *labia majora*. The *clitoris* is situated where the *labia minora* meet at the front, and is the most sensitive part of all.

The Clitoris
Although it is only 1 centimetre long, the clitoris is richly supplied with nerve endings and packs into its small size as much feeling as a man's penis. It also has the same trick of going hard when it is stimulated.

The area between the *labia* is called the *vestibule*. From front to back it houses the exit of the *urethra* (the tube carrying urine from the bladder) and the entrance to the vagina. The back edge of the vagina is bounded by the *perineum*, a small area of tissue which gets stretched – and sometimes torn – during labour. Further to the rear is the *anus*, the way out for solid waste from the digestive system.

Internal Arrangements

The Vagina
This runs from the outside to the womb, and is about 10 cm (4 ins) long. It is a muscular tube with a smooth lining, which normally lies flat. The *cervix*, meaning neck, is the entrance to the womb. It projects into the upper part of the vagina at an angle, but in older people it does not stick out so much.

The Womb, or Uterus
This is a container which is mainly muscle. It is 7.5 cm (3 ins) long and its walls are 2 cm thick. It leans forward from the vagina in most people, but it is not unusual or abnormal for it to be angled backwards. The womb is then said to be *retroverted* (back-leaning). The cervix takes up about a third of the womb's length and is narrower than the main body of the organ.

The Fallopian Tubes
The upper two-thirds of the womb are wedge-shaped, the widest part uppermost, with two corners like ears. From each of these a narrow tube stretches outwards and upwards, reaching out to the ovary on each side. Each tube ends in a frilly funnel to catch the eggs that are released from the ovary when they are mature enough to be fertilized. The ovaries, tubes, uterus and vagina are supported by ligaments – broad ribbons of fibrous tissue.

The Ovaries
These are storehouses for the materials from which future generations can develop. They are two solid, almond-shaped bodies, 2 cm by 2.5 across and 1 cm thick. During the reproductive period (puberty to the menopause) the ovaries contain *follicles*, each containing an egg-cell. When a follicle is ripe – that is, mature – it pops and the egg-cell, or *ovum*, falls into the conveniently placed Fallopian tube. It is then conveyed along this tube to the womb.

   After around age 40, most women have had the children they want – and can cope with – and the production of new eggs slows down. After the menopause, the ovaries become smaller and some of their hormonal work is taken over by the nearby adrenal glands.

Neighbours of the Genital System

Important structures in the locality of the genital system include the two cleansing and waste-disposal departments – the urinary system and the colon, rectum and anus. The bladder lies behind the pubic bone, between it and the womb. The narrow urine tube, the urethra, runs to the surface to come out just in front of the vagina, while two even smaller tubes, the *ureters*, bring the urine to the bladder from the kidneys. The ureters hug the side of the womb and can be pressed upon by, for instance, the presence of a large fibroid.

The waste-disposal unit for the motions lies behind the ovaries, womb and vagina and is separated from them by the perineal body, consisting of flexible packing. Two broad, flat sheets of muscle, the *levators*, support the three holes: the urethra, the vagina, and the anus – and the relevant organs. It is these muscles that you learn to exercise if you have trouble with leaks of urine – a common problem for women of 50-plus.

Lymph nodes in the groin and sites nearby provide a first-aid system for dealing with germs and cancer cells from the genital system by catching and detaining them before they reach the bloodstream. The nodes or glands then become swollen and, in the case of an infection, tender.

This, then, is the apparatus that is involved in the changes of the menopause. It can be useful to familiarize yourself with it, as this will help you understand the changes you will be going through in the menopause.

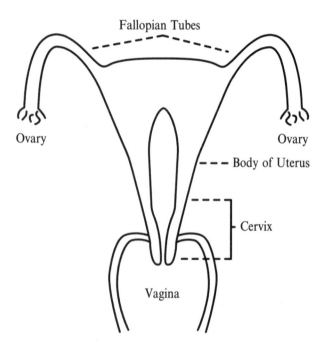

Diagram of Genital System

Chapter 3

How the System Works: The Controls

The genital system, like your digestive, urinary and circulatory systems, comes under the overriding control of the pituitary gland, in association with the hypothalamus, in the centre of your brain. Although the pituitary is only the size of a pea – and the same shape – it acts like the conductor of an orchestra. It keeps the various parts of your body working together harmoniously, each with its individual timing. For example, your heart keeps beating between 50 and 100 times a minute, you sleep around 8 hours in every 24, and during the reproductive years there is a monthly cycle of activity involving your womb and ovaries.

The Pituitary Hormones

The mechanism of control is by hormones: chemicals manufactured by your pituitary gland and hypothalamus, and released into the bloodstream. The hypothalamus contains a timing device called the 'pulse generator' which organizes the rate of release of the hormones. Rather like the postal system, these hormones, travelling with many others all round your body, convey messages to specific organs as though they were addressed to them. Important hormones in the control of the genital system are:

FSH, follicle-stimulating hormone
LH, luteinizing hormone

FSH and LH, in conjunction, activate the ovaries. FSH, as its name suggests, is responsible for the development of the follicles which contain the egg-cells, or *ova*. A surge of LH gives the go-ahead for ovulation, the release of an egg-cell. FSH in particular also stimulates the ovaries to produce the two female sex hormones: oestrogen and progesterone.

FSH and LH are of special interest when you are approaching menopause age and want to check whether you are indeed beginning the change. For example, flooding or irregular periods may be caused by other conditions, which call for treatment. Examples include fibroids, polyps, endometriosis (overgrowth of the lining of the womb) or possibly a tumour. A high level of FSH and LH in the blood indicates that the ovary is not responding to stimulation and that ovulation has not occurred at the

13

usual time. The likeliest cause is that the ovaries are running short of egg-cells – the first hint of the process leading to the menopause.

The Sex Hormones

Oestrogen – What It Does for You
- It is responsible for your sexual development at puberty.
- It maintains the structure and health of your sex organs – the uterus, tubes and vagina, and also the breasts.
- It does the same thing for the urine tube (the urethra) and the sensitive part of the bladder (the trigone), which alerts you when you need to pass water.
- All these parts only work comfortably, for instance for sex, with some lubrication, which is also due to oestrogen.
- It keeps up the supply of collagen to keep your skin supple and ward off dryness and wrinkles.
- It stimulates the uptake of calcium by your bones, protecting them against osteoporosis.
- It maintains the health of your joint surfaces, keeping the wear-and-tear disorder, osteoarthritis, at bay.
- It checks the amount of fat in your blood, making furred-up arteries and a heart attack less likely.
- It has a direct effect on the walls of the blood vessels, so that they retain their elasticity and allow the maximum amount of oxygen to be carried to the tissues. This is of particular importance to your brain and your heart, reducing the risks of stroke and heart attack.
- It increases the amount of protein in your body, but it has far less muscle-building effect than the male hormones (androgens).
- It maintains your feminine figure – not only your breasts but the layer of fat over your hips, bottom and thighs. Women often want to minimize this, but to men it is a turn-on.
- Last but not least, oestrogen increases your mental and physical energy and enhances a feeling of optimism. This is similar to the upbeat mood which often occurs in the first fortnight of your menstrual cycle.

Progesterone
This is far less important than oestrogen, though it works with oestrogen in protecting your bones from osteoporosis. It has the beneficial effect of pepping up your immune system and it is also mildly calming. In the peri-menopause, when ovulation is becoming less frequent, the ovaries make less progesterone and this can lead to heavy or unpredictable periods.

Testosterone
This male hormone is produced in small quantities in the ovaries and adrenal glands, and spices up the hormonal mix. It is responsible for libido in both sexes. After the change the ovaries produce more testosterone, but they also develop the knack of converting it into oestrogen, compensating to some degree for the reduction in supplies.

Alternative Sources of Oestrogen
The ovaries, stimulated by the pituitary hormones, provide nearly all your oestrogen from puberty to the change. When you are nudging 40, its production begins to fall off, although your periods are still regular. There are fewer follicles for ripening, but the process is so gradual that for several years after your last period your ovaries will still be making a significant amount of oestrogen.

Until then a small amount of oestrogen is made by the adrenal glands, which sit on top of the kidneys. As your need for an alternative supply of oestrogen develops, this supply increases. Another source of oestrogen is testosterone, and particularly its derivative androstenedione, which is also made by the adrenals. Helped by the liver, body fat can also be used to make oestrone, a weak form of oestrogen. Plump women sail through the menopause years with minimal signs of lack of oestrogen – most obviously, their complexions remain youthful.

Other Factors Affecting Oestrogen Supplies
- Your emotions: stress and distress cut production, while happy, warm feelings tend to increase it.
- Either an overactive or underactive thyroid gland may lead to interference with the production of oestrogen.
- Diet has a profound effect on oestrogen manufacture. Oestrogen levels are reduced in dedicated slimmers, anorexics and people suffering from debilitating illnesses, all of whom are underweight. Conversely, to be overweight is a plus in terms of keeping up your oestrogen supply.

Chapter 4

Symptoms and Signs: Local

Some women sail through their 40s and wake up one morning to a date ringed on their calendar and find that the expected period has not arrived. And never does. This is their menopause.

Only a small minority reach it in this non-event way, however. Four out of five of us have at least some of the symptoms heralding the change. And those who have an earlier-than-usual menopause, for whatever reason, tend to have especially severe menopausal symptoms. Whenever they occur, these symptoms may include disrupted, irregular or painful periods, vaginal changes, prolapse of the womb, urinary problems, changes to the skin and hair, bone, muscle or joint pain, bowel problems, changes to the breasts, and even more pronounced pre-menstrual syndrome (PMS) symptoms than you have experienced before.

Disrupted Periods

The essence of the menopause is the cessation of the periods, and the most obvious sign that this is on the cards is a faltering in the regular monthly cycle. Two aspects are affected: the timing and the flow.

Typically, the irregular cycle runs initially from 28 days to as little as 21 days. Later on the cycle becomes extra long and, increasingly, periods are skipped. When this happens, especially the first time, you may think you are pregnant. Occasionally you are right.

Warning
Although there are far fewer egg-cells left in your ovaries, from time to time one will be released – making a pregnancy possible. You need to continue with contraception for at least 18 months after your periods begin losing their rhythm. The combined oral contraceptive pill – with oestrogen and progesterone – is a good choice in the run-up to the menopause. It is 95% effective and has the additional benefit of offering some protection against heavy, irregular bleeding, fibroids, non-cancerous lumpy breasts, PMS and also the long-term risks of cancer of the womb or ovary.

Regular But Unduly Heavy Periods

These are nearly always due to the upset in the hormonal controls, particularly in late starters.

Irregular Periods

These are normal in the menopause, but irregular bleeding between periods, after intercourse or when it is more than a year since your last period needs looking into. It is likely to be due to one of the disorders of the womb such as fibroids, endometriosis, an infection or, rarely, a cancer.

Painful Periods (Dysmenorrhoea)

This is common when your periods are starting up, but can also occur at this stage, when they are bowing out. The cause will be in the womb or vagina. The immune system is less efficient in the menopause, so an infection can arise more easily.

The Vagina

The mucous glands which lubricate the lining of the vagina become reduced in number in reaction to the reduction in oestrogen in the area. This can mean that the lining of the vagina – and also of the cervix and uterus – becomes thinner and dryer. *Dyspareunia* – painful sexual intercourse – is one result of this.

Case Study

Helen and Bob got married when they were in their early 50s. They had both been through previous marriages and had children who were now grown up. They did not want any more children, but they did want to enjoy a normal sex life. It was a terrible disappointment to Helen when she found the process far from pleasurable, even excruciating. Ordinary lubricants like KY jelly brought some relief, but what really saved the situation was an oestrogen cream. Helen had been hesitant about starting on HRT – as she'd been so glad she no longer had to take the contraceptive pill every day. The vaginal problem helped her to take the plunge, however. The oestrogen cream was messy and not suitable for indefinite use; HRT tablets worked equally well. Another help was the beneficial effect of practice. Neither Bob nor Helen had been having regular intercourse while they were without partners, but once Helen's vaginal dryness was overcome the regular love-making stimulated her remaining mucous glands.

Sometimes vaginal dryness leads to bleeding or infection. The latter is more likely when the lining is thinner and more fragile, and also because the vaginal discharge becomes less acid around the menopause. This, in turn, discourages the friendly *Döderlein's bacillus*, which protects the vagina from other bacteria. Acetic acid gel (brand name Aci-jel), inserted once or twice a day, is helpful when infection is a problem. If the discharge, instead of being clear and watery, is thick and creamy, yellow, green or frothy, this indicates that one of the common vaginal infections has taken hold and will require the appropriate drug treatment.

While such infections often come through intercourse, during the menopause (when the immune system is not working to full efficiency) vaginal infections can crop up in women who have had no recent sexual activity.

Another effect of the change is a slight shortening of the vagina, though not enough to interfere with your sexual enjoyment, and a reduction in size of the cervix and womb – a sensible adjustment when there is no longer a need for them to be able to expand to accommodate a growing foetus.

Prolapse of the Womb

The ligaments which support your vagina and womb lose some of their strength with the approach of the menopause, especially if they have been over-stretched in the past by having babies. With less oestrogen the tissues lose some of their elasticity and the weight of the womb can drag it down into the vagina. This is called *prolapse*. Sometimes a pouch of vaginal skin, including some bladder, bulges into the vagina – this is called a *cystocoele*. Less often, something similar occurs involving a fold of rectum protruding into the vagina – a *rectocoele*.

Either of these loose pouches of vaginal skin can press on the urethra and cause or worsen a leakage of urine – urinary incontinence (see below). A rectocoele can also interfere with your passing a motion. In these cases sometimes pelvic muscle exercises help, and HRT also helps, but if the symptoms are really troublesome a surgical repair can revolutionize a woman's life.

The Urinary System

Your water system is closely associated with the genital system. The membrane lining the bladder and the urethra, like that inside the vagina and uterus, is affected by the shortage of oestrogen.

Cystitis
When the membrane lining the bladder and urethra becomes thinner and

more liable to breakdown, this can let infection in, so that cystitis (inflammation of the bladder) becomes more common after the menopause. It is estimated to affect more than 10% of women over 60. One way to combat it is to make your urine more alkaline by drinking water with sodium bicarbonate in it. Cranberry juice has the same effect and is much more pleasant to drink. An opposite treatment is to increase the acidity of the vagina to encourage the protective bacilli. Coffee and alcohol should be avoided, as both irritate the bladder. An oestrogen cream in the vagina is another approach, but if the symptoms continue, a urine test followed by whichever antibiotic is appropriate will deal with any infection.

The Urethral Syndrome
The typical symptoms of cystitis include frequency of passing water, with pain or burning, but in half the women of menopausal age who have these symptoms there is no evidence of infection. The most common cause is vaginitis (inflammation of the vagina), also affecting the urethra, the opening of which is next to that of the vagina. It is not germs but cracks in the lining of the urethra and the vagina due to dryness from lack of oestrogen that are responsible.

Itching round the vaginal opening, and sometimes also that of the urethra, can be unbearably irritating, especially as it is not an area where you want to be seen rubbing or scratching yourself. Sometimes it is as severe as pain. The treatment is an oestrogen cream applied to both openings two or three times a day: Premarin or Dienoestrol creams are equally effective. The clue that tells you that this is not cystitis is that the pain or discomfort is all on the outside, for instance there is no lower abdominal pain.

Urinary Incontinence
The trigone, the doorkeeper to the bladder, become thinner and more sensitive in the change. You may find that you need to pass water more frequently and that it is difficult to wait.

Urge incontinence is an involuntary leakage of urine when you suddenly want to pass water and cannot get to the loo in time.

Case Study
Joanna was bugged by this embarrassing problem, although she was only 56, by no stretch of the imagination 'old'. She found her woman doctor sympathetic and helpful. She explained that the trigone could become extra sensitive as part of the change and this, coupled with the muscles becoming weaker over time, could impair Joanna's control. She referred her to the district nurse attached to the practice, who taught Joanna how to strengthen her muscles through exercise.

KEGEL EXERCISES (devised by Dr Arnold Kegel)
Stop the flow when you are in the middle of passing water. This will involve the sphincter muscle (the one that closes off the bladder) and enables you to feel its action.

1. Tighten your sphincter muscle, hold for 3 full seconds (a second is a count of 4), then release for 1 second. Repeat 6 times, 3 times a day. Or try version 2:
2. Contract the sphincter for 1 second, relax for one second – repeat 20 times, also 3 times a day.
3. Hold the contraction for 10 full seconds, then relax for 5 seconds. Repeat 5 times, 3 times a day.

Joanna could only do the third version when she had already practised the other two for about 10 days.

THE VAGINAL CONE
This is another type of exercise aimed at strengthening the pelvic muscles. A series of weighted plastic cones are inserted into the vagina and you have to try and hold them in, starting with the lightest.
    Joanna tried this method, too. She found the effect of the exercises helped her considerably with control of her bladder, and as an added bonus it enhanced her satisfaction in sexual intercourse.

Oestradiol Pessaries (Vagifem)
Another treatment for incontinence is to insert oestrogen pessaries into the vagina once or twice a day for two to three months.

Stress Incontinence
This somewhat different from the urge type of difficulty. It means a leakage of urine when you cough, laugh or run, for instance while playing sport. The same treatments can be applied (i.e. the Kegel exercises and vaginal cone), but they may not be as effective as in urge incontinence, and it is sometimes worthwhile to have an operation to strengthen and support the neck of the bladder. This operation is called colporrhaphy (kolpos - vagina/rhaphe - sewing, in Greek).

Changes in the Skin and Hair

Like the lining membranes of the sexual organs, during the perimenopause your skin becomes thinner and drier. You never see a menopausal woman with coarse, greasy or spotty skin. It is more delicate, and looks more attractive, sometimes almost transparent, but bruises easily, partly because the blood vessels underneath are also more fragile. This is the time when your skin will really benefit from moisturizing creams and lotions. They act by smoothing the surface and increasing the water content by preventing its loss into the air. Aqueous cream BP is as good as any, simple and reasonably priced. You can use it in place of soap to wash your face.

What is even more important, however, is to avoid the things which damage your skin: coffee, alcohol, nicotine and exposure to the sun. Between them they can age your skin 10 years ahead of the rest of you.

In the 10 years following the menopause your skin can lose up to 30% of its collagen, the connective tissue which supports it and makes it tough and flexible. Losing collagen ultimately leads to wrinkles, but HRT checks this trend within a few months through special oestrogen receptors in the deeper layers of the skin.

Case Study
Debbie resented the whole idea of the change, interpreting it as a doom-laden pathway to getting, and looking, old and unsexy rather than the entrance to a new, more free era of life. At first she simply plastered more make-up on her face, but the lines and sags showed through. She decided on drastic action. She discarded the idea of having a skin peel – the effect is only temporary and not radical enough. She went for an expensive full face-lift with collagen implants round the eyes.

It was a pity her neck, eyes and hands were such a give-away, and of course she would need a few more tucks after about five years – and the repeats are never as good as the first one. Skin that is stimulated by outdoor exercise and adequately moisturized looks fresh and healthy, and an interest in other people makes it look charming to them.

Your Hair
Just as your skin becomes finer and drier, so does your hair. You will not have lank, greasy hair but it may be weaker and thinner, and difficult to manage. As with your skin, this is the time when conditioners and thickeners come into their own. Your skin, hair and nails will all benefit from a little cossetting. Because your skin and hair are more delicate than before, avoid harsh soaps and detergents; wash your hair frequently but use the mildest shampoo; protect it and your skin from direct sunlight, and use a bathing cap if you are swimming in chlorinated water. It is a matter of health, not vanity.

While it is oestrogen that keeps your hair strong, it is the male hormones, the androgens, that are responsible for its growth. When you have less oestrogen available, the small amount of androgen you make becomes relatively more important. This can have the effect of making your hair thinner in the parts where men become bald, and can also lead to a small increase in the amount of hair on your face. Your pubic hair – though relatively unimportant – also diminishes after the menopause.

Your nails become more brittle with the reduction in collagen, but if they have longitudinal ridges it means that you are short of iron: this is common at this stage in life, but easily corrected with iron tablets.

Sore Eyes
This is part of the dryness syndrome. If your eyes are too dry they may feel as though you have grit in them, especially in the morning, when you first open them. There are useful over-the-counter preparations you can buy: artificial tears – hypromellose eye drops, to use as needed during the day – and a soft clear paraffin ointment (Lacri-lube) to put in for the night. Your eyes, from being uncomfortably sore, will adjust after a few weeks' treatment, and then require less and less – but you cannot give it up altogether.

Dry Throat and Mouth
More of the same syndrome, these are often made worse by medicines such as antidepressants or water tablets. Sucking lemon drops and frequent small drinks are a help. Alcohol makes matters worse – it is water the tissues are thirsty for. They are missing the effect of oestrogen in stimulating the blood supply and the amount of water in the surface tissues – the skin and membranes.

Bones, Muscles and Joints

Collagen is the connective and 'packing' material which supports all the other tissues, including the muscles, joints and bones. The strength and resilience of your bones depends, not on calcium, valuable though it is, but on collagen. Collagen production is stimulated by oestrogen, so at the menopause, when there is less oestrogen, your bones keep their size and shape but become brittle. This is part of osteoporosis.

Your joints depend on collagen even more than the bones, to protect the joint surfaces from grating and shock. Osteoarthritis, joint damage from wear and tear, affects everyone over 35 to some extent, but it tends to escalate at the menopause. Oestrogen therapy, HRT, works wonders by checking bone turnover and allowing collagen to build up, however severe the damage.

Health-food shops sell glucosamine and chondroitin, which are meant to nourish the gristly parts (the collagen) of the joints, and some people find these tablets helpful. They certainly do no harm. The other treatments are graduated exercises, anti-inflammatory pain-killing medicines (NSAIDs) and physiotherapy. Joint and muscle pain, which our grand-mothers lumped together as 'rheumatism', are common in the meno-pause, as part of the general changes going on in your body.

Your Bowels

The constipation which commonly crops up in the perimenopause is part of the general trend to dryness. If you have not already prepared for this, you must increase the natural fibre in your diet and the amount of water you drink, and do exercises that work your abdominal muscles.

Breast Changes

Oestrogen was responsible for the development of your breasts in early adolescence. After the menopause they become smaller – an advantage for some of us. The nipples are less prominent and the skin around them darkens slightly, as it does in pregnancy. This is an age when regular self-examination and mammograms are important, to nip in the bud any pos-sibility of a cancer, but the menopausal lack of oestrogen is not a risk factor.

PMS: The Premenstrual Syndrome

This syndrome, with its many assorted symptoms, is one you can expect to be rid of after your menopause. Unfortunately, in the latter part of the run-up to that event, when your hormone levels are fluctuating, PMS can become even more troublesome, or start up for the first time. A dip in the progesterone level in particular can trigger an attack, while progesterone and water tablets (diuretics) are used to treat it, together with counselling if you have distressing mood changes.

The symptoms include physical ones such as backache and pelvic dis-comfort, sore breasts, bloating and water retention, as well as headaches and irritability – even leading some women to violence. PMS, like the menopause, affects every system of the body.

Chapter 5

Symptoms and Signs: General

The most common indications of the change, and those which are the subject of the bitterest complaints, are the so-called *vasomotor* symptoms. 'Vaso' refers to blood vessels, in this case in the skin, and 'motor' means the only movements they are capable of – constricting and dilating.

There are three key vasomotor symptoms:
- hot flushes
- night sweats
- palpitations.

No one fully understands the mechanism for these symptoms, but the top theory is that the temperature-control centre in the hypothalamus is put out of action by varying hormone levels, with the lack of oestrogen being of key importance. The small blood vessels to the skin dilate, making it feel hot, and this may in turn induce sweating.

Hot Flushes

These are especially unpleasant, coming on suddenly without warning, and often embarrassingly noticeable to other people. Usually the flush starts with a feeling of pressure in your head, then heat and redness rise rapidly up your neck and face into your scalp, spread to your chest and shoulders and finally involve your whole body. The whole episode may last only a matter of seconds – or can be as long as 15 minutes, recurring several times a day. It is often accompanied by sweating, a rapid, thumping heart beat and a sense of panic.

Case Study
Susie was typical. Her hot flushes started when she was 47. At first they occurred only in the week before a period, but gradually became more frequent and unpredictable. Aside from what her hormones were doing, Susie found several triggers which would bring on a flush, for instance a hot curry, or coffee, tea or alcohol. Most potent of all, was anxiety or embarrassment – or even the enjoyable stimulus of entertaining friends to a meal. It reminded her of the shyness and blushing she had endured in her teens.

As the flush faded, Susie would feel deadly cold and shivery, yet sweaty at the same time. While Susie said the sensation of flushing was like a flame running over her skin, some of her friends likened it to having hot oil sprayed on their faces.

Night Sweats

Apart from hot or cold sweats and a fast heart rate coming on as part of the flush, episodes of severe sweating often occur in the small hours: night sweats. They usually follow the same time-scale as the flushes, increasing in the perimenopause, then gradually becoming infrequent.

Palpitations

The opening up of the blood vessels and the feeling of heat induce a speed-up of your heart rate, of which you are uncomfortably aware. It may be coupled with a feeling of faintness and general weakness.

The whole vasomotor syndrome, or parts of it, usually continues for two or three years, but if the symptoms begin early, for instance when you are just 40, they may go on for as long as 10 years, although becoming less severe. A quarter to a half of menopausal women have occasional flushes more than five years after the start of the menopause.

Although the vasomotor group is the most important, a range of other, disparate symptoms are commonly ascribed to the menopause. They include:

● Headaches
● Neck and backache
● Difficulty sleeping
● Weight gain
● Feelings in the skin of numbness, tingling or a weird crawling sensation
● Bloating of the abdomen
● Breast discomfort or pain
● Fatigue without cause.

There are also a number of emotional, mind and mood changes – these are discussed in Chapter 6.

Coping with Menopausal Symptoms

The explanation of the symptoms is bound up with the sex hormones, and the gold standard treatment is HRT. However, some women cannot take

HRT, and it is not 100% effective, especially for hot flushes.

Other Methods

Some of these seem almost as unacceptable as cupping and bleeding. Cupping is a method of drawing blood to the surface of the skin by pressing a hollow vessel onto it and causing suction. Some women have been recommended the renunciation, for life, of coffee, tea, chocolate, alcohol, sugar, salt – plus, of course, tobacco. Plenty of filtered water is allowed. Other suggested methods include hypnotherapy (including self-hypnosis), a DIY method that is easy to learn.

The British Medical Association's Tips
- Avoid hot food and drinks, coffee, alcohol and spices, or eating in the late evening.
- Avoid anxiety and other stress – easier said, but at least you can postpone some events, like moving house.
- Wear clothing in loose, thin layers, made of natural fibres such as pure cotton.
- Cotton sheets.
- Cool bedroom.
- Take lukewarm showers instead of soaking in a hot bath.
- Relaxation exercises from your GP, practice nurse or physiotherapist.
- Take vitamin E and Evening Primrose Oil supplements.
- Eat soya-based dishes, since soya is a rich source of phyto-oestrogens, the oestrogen-like compounds found in plants. Ginseng is similar, and other herbs have been used for centuries to relieve menopausal symptoms, for instance Motherwort and raspberry leaf tea, Lady's Mantle and Agnus castus (see also Chapter 15).

Chapter 6

Psychological and Emotional Effects

When something strange is happening to your body, in the part that is inextricably bound up with your thinking and feeling – the genital or reproductive system – it is inevitable that you should react psychologically. There is an upheaval in your sex hormones, with the change in emphasis from preparing for a possible pregnancy every month to running the system smoothly and economically and allowing you the freedom to do what you like when you like, unencumbered.

The change from regular periods to none at all is usually spread over two years or more, and proceeds unevenly – more like climbing a rocky hillside than walking sedately along a path. You may hardly notice the start – mild swings of mood without apparent cause over as long as 10 years – well before you are even thinking of the change. The impact comes with the first definite indication that it is approaching. It may be a very light or an unduly heavy period, or one that comes out of sequence. Your immediate reaction will affect how you cope in the coming months and how troublesome you will find any symptoms.

If you are self-confident and secure in your sense of personal worth, any symptoms will be pinpricks of little significance. However, 99% of us are not so carefree about navigating uncharted waters.

Loss of Self-esteem

Case Study
Rachel was 48 when her periods started playing up. She had an orderly mind and liked her life to run to a routine. Her work in the accounts department of a big hardware chain suited her admirably, and she prided herself on her efficiency. She was thrown when she found that she could no longer plan her favourite walking holidays when she could be certain of avoiding a period. Then, to her horror, she started making silly, but fortunately unimportant mistakes, in much the same way as sometimes happens with a period or during pregnancy.

Rachel's concentration was slipping, her memory, usually spot-on, let her down once or twice, and her attention span had shrunk to that of a two-year-old. The result was a disastrous loss of self-esteem. This is a common reaction to the menopause, and it is not improved by the sexist/ageist stigma that still attaches to this phase of a woman's life. 'Menopausal' is used as a disparaging term, usually by those men who conveniently ignore their own andropause.

It is difficult in the face of this to remember that around age 50 a woman is at the height of her intellectual powers, has mastered her social skills and garnered a body of experience and hard knowledge. Her physical health is at a high point, and her looks reflect this. Logically, her self-esteem should be at its peak.

Sense of Loss

There are gains from the menopause, but all change involves some losses, and it is these that often dominate a woman's thoughts at this time.

- Loss of the ability to have babies – even if she would be horrified to find herself pregnant.
- Loss of sexual attractiveness – this is only in the woman's mind – most men judge it by the packaging, while charm means someone who is interested in them.
- Loss of femininity – as above. The ovaries go on producing the sex hormones for years after the last period, and by then the compensatory mechanisms are in place. Besides, it is mainly a matter of the image a woman chooses to present.
- Loss of her figure: this is something you can alter if you put your mind to it, but there are plenty of well-dressed, dynamic women who are a few pounds overweight.
- Loss of career possibilities – but there are courses galore to widen your knowledge, and less difficulty than ever before in landing a new job as a mature, reliable person.
- Loss of youth – with the spectres of old age and feeble health – when you can look forward to over a decade of particularly good health.

The Bereavement Syndrome

If you feel that the menopause means that you have lost something precious, including your role in life, your mind may react as though you have lost a loved one. The various stages of bereavement are:

1. Denial – you refuse to believe that the tell-tale signs – disrupted periods and hot flushes – can possibly mean you are into the menopause.
2. Sadness – weepiness takes over, and often you become anxious and restless. You eat and sleep badly and feel that somehow you are at fault. This stage can last for weeks.
3. Acceptance – the reality of the menopause slowly sinks in.

Case Study
Barbara had married late, to a widower with two children. At 45 she still hoped that she and Jeff would have a baby and that she would go through the experience of motherhood. She had more reason than most to reject the idea of the change, but hormone tests showed a very high FSH level, indicating that her ovaries were no longer producing eggs. She plunged into a bereavement reaction when the situation was explained to her. She blamed herself bitterly because she had not tried for a baby earlier, although it had not been possible for her. She brooded over the matter constantly.

Barbara might have fallen into a clinical depression but for the needs of Jeff's children. Over time she became convinced that she was 'meant' to be free to look after them, and built a warm, loving relationship with them.

Case Study
Genevieve stopped at the denial stage. She simply would not accept that she was menopausal. In fact, she fought the concept head on:
● She wore her skirts shorter and tighter than ever, although her legs were not wonderful, and her decolletage was more revealing than ever.
● She tortured her hair by the generous application of dye.
● She flirted inappropriately with any man, however young.
● She had her one grandchild call her Genevieve rather than Grandma.
● She lied blatantly about her age and struggled to forget the music and films that she should not have been able to remember.

The trouble was Genevieve deceived no one, not even herself in her heart of hearts. Her family found her behaviour acutely embarrassing, and it was fortunate that she could not keep it up. The bonus was that she retained her interest, though slightly toned down, in her appearance, and put a cheerful gloss on whatever was happening. She also kept up with the activities she enjoyed – swimming, the theatre and socialising.

Anxiety

Anxiety is a common, understandable reaction to the menopause.

Case Study
Lucy had a reasonably interesting job in the Health Service, a steady if unexciting husband, and two children just starting out in life. There were no serious financial or health problems, but at the first sign of the menopause Lucy became anxious. It affected her physically:
● She took hours to get to sleep, however exhausted, and sometimes she

would wake several times in the night, before being roused by the alarm, unwilling and unrefreshed.

- Lack of sleep left her tired during the day, but she could not relax.
- She did not lose her appetite, as happens to many sufferers from anxiety, but found herself eating compulsively, without enjoyment. Nothing had any taste.
- She had to go to the loo to pass water half a dozen times a day, and was plagued with frequent urgent, loose motions.
- Her muscles ached, all over her body. This was because they were at greater tension than usual, although she did not realize it.
- Another change of which Lucy was only vaguely aware was her increased heart rate – this was one of the causes of her feeling exhausted – for no reason, as it seemed to her.

She kept getting waves of anxiety, but not about anything specific that she could have dealt with.

Lucy struggled on her own for some weeks, telling herself not to be so stupid, but finally she consulted her GP. He gave her a choice between tablets and counselling, and she chose the latter. Some people need both, but unhurried discussion slowly defused her anxiety, helped by the gradual stabilization of her chaotic hormones.

Depressed Mood

This occurs as often as anxiety during the menopause, affecting at least 60% of women. It is not the same as a clinical depression, with its deadening of all vitality, but comprises a mood of sadness, often with tears.

Case Study
Cynthia was only 46 when her periods stopped abruptly.

- She felt cheated that 'all the good part of her life was over.'
- She could only envisage a steady decline ahead.
- She was, she felt, no use to anyone now.
- She often cried in private, and even in public Cynthia was a miserable companion, seeing only the down side.
- Her food brought no pleasure, although she ate it automatically.
- She refused so many invitations that her friends got tired of asking her.
- She had no patience with or interest in the activities of her children, her friends, her work colleagues or her husband.

Cynthia did recover after several wretched months, greatly helped by HRT and the understanding of her family.

Irritability

A short fuse is a characteristic symptom of the menopause. A normally considerate woman can act in ways that are completely out of character, becoming snappy with her nearest and dearest, her friends and her work colleagues. Everything seems to conspire to frustrate her. Her reactions are often associated with anxiety, and treatments that help alleviate anxiety may help with this symptom as well.

Panic Attacks

These frequently crop up for the first time during the menopause. Statistically they are three times as common in women as men. They comprise sudden bursts of acute anxiety which build up rapidly, with a range of physical symptoms. These will include some, but not all, of the following:
- Flushes or chills
- Shortness of breath and a feeling of being suffocated
- Choking
- Palpitations – which may bring on the fear of having a heart attack
- Pain or tightness in the chest, which reinforces this fear
- Fear of death or of going mad
- Sweating
- Dizziness
- Feeling of faintness
- Nausea and stomach pain
- Uncontrollable trembling
- Numbness or tingling in the hands or round the mouth
- A weird feeling of being detached from your body.

Hyperventilation

Hyperventilation means rapid, shallow breathing – sometimes complicating a panic attack. It washes the carbon dioxide out of your bloodstream, causing dizziness, ringing in the ears, headache and muscle spasms in the hands and feet.

Benzodiazepine medicines likeValium can control panic attacks, but are addictive. Some antidepressants help the symptoms. For an attack of hyperventilation the immediate cure is to breathe in and out of a paper bag, and in the longer term being taught better breathing techniques.

Agoraphobia

A surprising number of those who suffer panic attacks in the menopause also develop agoraphobia. It usually originates in a particular episode, for example in the queue for a bus or at the supermarket checkout. The sufferer suddenly panics without knowing why, feels faint and has alarming palpitations. After that she feels anxious whenever she feels trapped somewhere, is in a crowd, or is away from home without anyone she knows. She knows it is unreasonable but cannot help her feeling, sometimes becoming acutely anxious merely thinking about a possible trip to the shops.

Once established, agoraphobia can go on for years. The treatment is similar to that for panic generally, but includes a form of therapy in which the sufferer is exposed to the situation she most fears, but has received training in coping with it and with her panicky feelings.

Loss of Libido

For some women the menopause, or the thought of its significance, turns off their sexual interest like a switch. This is independent of the understandable turn-off when intercourse is uncomfortable because of dryness of the vagina. Quite a lot of women give up sexual intercourse at this time, although with the help of the contraceptive Pill and HRT there is no physical reason not to enjoy it for many years after the menopause – to the benefit of the organs concerned (see also pp 106-110).

Depressive Illness

A clinical depression, unlike a depressed mood, is rare in the menopause. It is the most serious reaction to the menopause, carrying with it the risk of suicide. To the sufferer the menopause means the snuffing out of all hope of having a child – a deadly blow to someone who cares about it deeply.

The Symptoms of Clinical Depression
- Low mood: a black cloud pervading everything with a sense of guilt
- Inability to raise any interest in your usual activities, and even the people you care about
- No concern for your appearance
- Pessimistic thoughts, always expecting the worst
- Drooping head and shoulders
- Poor concentration and memory
- Difficulty in making decisions

- Loss of appetite, leading to weight loss
- Early waking, two or three hours earlier than normal. This is the worst part of the day.
- Loss of energy, being easily fatigued but vaguely restless
- A slowing down in thought and speech
- Constipation

No one has all these symptoms, but three or four are enough to tell you that this is more than ordinary sadness.

The treatment includes antidepressant medication, usually one of the selective serotonin re-uptake inhibitors (SSRIs) in the Prozac group. Cognitive psychotherapy, a talking treatment, is the other main treatment.

External Causes of Depression and Anxiety

The menopause years, 45 to 55, come along at a time in most women's lives when there are changes quite apart from the hormonal ones. Some upsetting life events and unwelcome situations are likely to crop up. Children leaving home can bring on the 'empty nest syndrome' – a feeling of loss and being no longer wanted, while your parents, too, are acquiring a different role in relation to you. There is a reversal of the years when they were the strong, knowledgeable ones from whom you could draw support. Now they have probably retired, slipping out of contact with your busy adult world. Their health may become a cause for concern, and one or other – usually the father – may die, putting you suddenly in the front line – the next generation to have to leave the stage.

Around now your face and figure may show unmistakeable signs of getting older. Your job may be on the line, because you no longer match the image of thrusting youth worshipped in our culture. It is also a critical stage for your marriage – or partnership. You are no longer building up a life together or centred around the children, so the marriage may seem to have lost its point. You partner, equally, may be searching for a fresh impetus and perhaps a tonic to his sex life – just when you are feeling disadvantaged in that area. It does not help that a generally depressive mood siphons off your vitality and makes you a dull companion.

Case Study
Astrid was 49, and wishing she could stick there. Arthur, her husband, had just been offered a prestigious post involving a lot of social engagements. Astrid's job, on the other hand, was chugging along much as usual, but with an influx of 'new blood' – a gaggle of ambitious 30-year-olds. Astrid was pleased for Arthur, and pleased for her son, David, that he had got the place he'd wanted at Aberdeen University. He was delighted to be going

to Scotland, and planned to stay there to do some hill-walking.

Astrid had been having a run of heavy periods and, without realizing it, had become anaemic. Her mood was subdued and she felt tired all the time. She found herself opting out of more and more of the dinners to which she was invited with Arthur. Her miserable emotional state was teetering on the borders of clinical depression when her friend, Rosemary, remarked that she looked washed out and bullied her into seeing the doctor. A six-week course of iron tablets, and Rosemary's support, helped Astrid to stop short of the brink of a depressive illness. With increasing energy – and looking better – she began to take more interest in the new people at work and in Arthur's colleagues and acquaintances.

Insomnia

While you are happily and peacefully slumbering your body repairs itself and your mind sorts the problems of the day into sense and order. How miserable it is, by contrast, if you cannot slip into sleep but toss about seemingly for hours, or you wake up tired but alert and find the clock says 2 or 3 a.m. and you cannot get back to sleep, either for ages or at all. You feel profoundly lonely with all the rest of the world unconscious.

Insomnia in the beginning, middle or late part of the night is one of the symptoms that can plague you around the menopause. It is most often due to the hormonal and emotional revolution that is going on inside you, or the physical aspects – hot flushes and night sweats. Sometimes it is part of an anxiety state or clinical depression.

What Can You Do About It?
1. Establish a bedtime ritual:
    - Establishing a regular bedtime, but not nursery hours. You are an adult, and if you try to sleep at 9.30 p.m., even if you succeed you will have slept out your deepest sleep by half-past midnight.
    - Have a small hot drink – milk or camomile tea, nothing with any caffeine in it – and teeth-cleaning.
    - Taking a warm bath.
    - Reading in bed, listening to the radio or watching TV for 20-30 minutes.
2. Have a warm, ventilated bedroom.
3. Do not have a late supper. Lying down with a full stomach is bad for your digestion and a strain on your heart.
4. Do not take stimulants in the evening such as coffee, tea or nicotine.
5. Be careful with alcohol – it may get you off to sleep, but it is metabolized away in an hour or two and you wake up, no longer sleepy.

6. Keep your fluids down in the evening, especially caffeine and alcohol, which stimulate the kidneys to make urine.
7. Take at least half-an-hour's exercise daily, preferably out of doors. Muscle tiredness is relaxing, unlike mental fatigue.
8. Check your sleeping arrangements – have you a sagging or uneven mattress, or a partner who snores?

Are your nights disturbed because of stress? If possible, deal with this before sleeptime.
   Common causes of stress, apart from the menopause itself:
   ● Work worries
   ● Relationship problems
   ● Bereavement and other losses
   ● Too much to do, too little time
   ● Changes – of place, job, role, such as becoming a grandparent
   ● Money worries.

Personality traits which cause stress: low self-confidence; short fuse; bossiness; tendency to give up; pessimistic outlook.

Stress Management through Relaxation
This is something you can do for yourself. Block off 15 minutes in warm, comfortable surroundings, lying down or well-supported in a chair.
● Focus your gaze on a mark on the ceiling or any other fixed point, or even an image in your mind.
● Breathe in and out slowly.
● Deliberately tense then relax one set of muscles after another, starting at your feet.
● Visualize a peaceful scene, such as clouds moving lazily across the sky, or imagine the sounds of breaking waves or the wind in the leaves.

Get up from your session relaxed, leaving your stress behind.

Chapter 7

Osteoporosis

Osteoporosis is a disease of the menopause. It can lead to long-term pain and crippling deformity because of bones that crumble or fracture. One in three of all women in the UK, the US and Australia will develop it at some time, and the odds shorten to one in two after the menopause. Fortunately there are precautions you can take in advance to prevent yourself becoming one of its victims. However, if you have not thought of it until now, and you are in the change, you should start on an anti-osteoporosis regime without delay. And at worst, if you already have some of the symptoms, there is a lot you can do to improve matters.

What Is Osteoporosis?

It is a weakening of the structure of the bones with a loss of the solid material, especially calcium. They can become so fragile that any knock or pressure may break them. Bones are not solid and homogenous like concrete, but living, changing, dynamic organs that are perpetually re-modelling themselves. There are two types of bone cell:

● Osteoclasts, which break down and remove worn-out bone. This is called *resorption*.
● Osteoblasts, the builders, molecule by molecule, of new, replacement tissue.

Bone itself comes in two forms: *cortical* and *trabecular*. The cortical bone makes up the impervious outer layer, like the bark of a tree, while, inside, the trabecular bone consists of soft fat and marrow within a honeycomb of strands of hard bone. The little bones of the spine, the vertebrae, are composed largely of trabecular bone, which makes them vulnerable to being crushed.

The Risk Factors in Osteoporosis

● General: the white races are more vulnerable than the black or brown, with the Scandinavians the most at risk – this is a matter of genetics. Living in Northern Europe or the United States also makes you more liable to develop osteoporosis. It is the relative lack of sunshine, with its power of enabling us to manufacture vitamin D in our skin, and hence absorb calcium, that underlies these differences.

- Personal genetics: a propensity to develop osteoporosis may be passed down to you in your genes. If any of your blood relatives have been sufferers, there is an increased risk – and a warning to take avoiding action. The strongest link is from mother to daughter.
- You have never had a child.
- You suffer from lactase deficiency, so that you cannot tolerate dairy products and do not take in enough calcium.
- Accidents involving injury to your bones.
- Irregular periods.
- Abdominal operations interfering with the absorption of calcium.
- Anorexia nervosa, severe slimming or other causes of malnutrition.

Looking After Your Bones

An absolute essential is to give up smoking, which brings forward the start of your menopause by about two years. HRT, or other forms of oestrogen, will not restore your bones if you smoke, as they would if you did not smoke.

Be moderate in your alcohol intake and keep within the 21-unit-a-week limit for women, and do not have more than five cups of coffee in the day – tea contains less caffeine and is also rich in antioxidants.

Regard over-the-counter drugs such as pain-killers, and especially recreational drugs, as potential poisons to your bones, and while you must take the medicines your doctor prescribes, remember that some of them will harm your bones, and try to keep to low doses. Steroids are the most dangerous to your bones, but others include thyroxine, anti-epileptics, heparin, lithium, major tranquillizers, aluminium (in indigestion mixtures), nitrites (for angina), theophylline (for asthma), and iron in excess.

Nourishment
A good, mixed, nutritious diet which provides plenty of dairy products and vitamins is as necessary for your bones as for your muscles, and it is safer to be slightly plump than very thin. If you fall and have no padding, your bones will take the brunt – and may break – but substantial overweight also throws a strain on them.

How Osteoporosis Shows Itself

Osteoporosis is often called 'the silent epidemic'. It affects vast numbers of people, but it develops so unobtrusively that you may not realize what is happening until some accident comes out of the blue and forces your attention. All the symptoms and signs come from breakages. The secret thief has been stealing the substance of your bones, making them increasingly fragile, since your early 40s. By the time you have had your last period and are well into your 50s, 20% of the minerals and protein of your bones will have gone – although their size and shape remain deceptively the same. It is like a house that was built of bricks and cement being replaced with one that looks the same, but is made of clay. Any jarring, stress or pressure will make it crack or crumble.

By 65 you will have lost twice as much bone substance, and by 75 you stand an even chance of already having experienced several compression fractures in your back. The odd twinge of backache may not have seemed remarkable enough to alert you to the situation.

The Effects of Fractured Vertebrae
The most obvious sign is your loss of height. You notice that cupboard shelves and coat hooks which used to be conveniently placed have mysteriously become out of reach, and it is difficult to sit or stand up straight.

Vertebral fractures come in two styles:
1. Incident: the bone gives way without warning when you cough or lift something heavy, or sit down or get up from a low chair. You feel something happen in your back – see below.
2. Prevalence type: these develop gradually, with no starting point that you can identify. They are caused little by little by the stresses of everyday movement, or the weight of the upper part of the body pressing down on your back.

Acute Symptoms of a Fractured Vertebra
- Pain in the area of the injured bone, sometimes spreading like a girdle round the trunk.
- Tenderness in the muscles lying over the fracture – they are in spasm in an effort to protect the injured part.
- Swelling.
- Impaired movements because of pain – more severe if you try bending, stooping or lifting.
- Colicky abdominal pain, with loss of appetite and sometimes vomiting.
- Fever.

Longer-term Effects
- Loss of height of more than 10 cm (4 ins) over a decade.
- Nipped nerve roots, because of the altered shape of the crushed

vertebrae, causing pain. This usually subsides spontaneously quite quickly.

- Numbness or paralysis from the same cause, and also likely to be temporary.
- Permanent stoop – the medical term is *kyphosis* and the folk description is 'dowager's hump'. It is not usually painful in itself but, coupled with a shortened back from the collapsed vertebrae, it may become impossible to expand your chest fully, so you become short of breath.
- It feels tiring to hold your head up, so when you are resting you are usually looking down.
- Balance disturbances: your balance may be upset by these changes, which affects your walking and standing, and makes you (understandably) afraid of falling over.
- Your lower ribs may rub against your hip bones as your back shrinks. This is usually more awkward than painful.
- Abdominal symptoms.

Case Study

Sarah was 70 before any symptoms she connected with osteoporosis cropped up. She knew she had lost height because she experienced difficulty reaching tins on the top shelves in her kitchen cupboards, and she noticed that it took a definite effort to hold her head and back erect. She did not realize at first that the symptoms in her abdomen were due to this same shortening of her body. She was puzzled – and rather annoyed – that although she was eating no more than usual, and in fact her weight remained steady at 8 stone (50.6 kg), her tummy was sticking out and she had no waist. It was the inevitable result of her abdomen having to accommodate itself to a space shorter by several inches, but not restricted forwards.

Another result of everything in Sarah's abdomen coming under pressure was constipation. She learned to take great care with her diet, drank plenty of liquids and used herbal laxatives when necessary, to ensure that her motions remained soft enough to pass easily. The added pressure on her bladder, combined with the long-term effects of having had four children and the weakening of the muscles involved, meant she had to pass water more often – or risk an embarrassing leakage. Care, pelvic exercises and the precautionary wearing of pads made her feel more secure.

None of Sarah's symptoms was painful or interfered with her way of living, but she was meticulous about taking calcium and fish-liver oil, and keeping to her daily 20- to 30-minute exercise session.

Hip Fractures

Twenty percent – 1 in 5 of women of 50-plus in the UK and US are is destined to have a hip fracture, compared with the 18% risk of a vertebral fracture. Sixty is the critical age. Falls become increasingly frequent from then, particularly if your balance has been disrupted by changes in your shape and height or the effects of another common disorder of middle age, osteoarthritis. Jarring your hip joint, for instance by stepping off the kerb rather suddenly, can be enough, while 5% of minor falls result in a hip fracture.

Usually you get no warning, but occasionally there is aching or a twinge of pain when you put weight on one side, for a few days or perhaps as long as a fortnight, before the break. If you are slim, your bones are less well padded – this increases the likelihood of fracture. The peak age for hip fracture is around 75, but it may happen in your 60s if there are extra risk factors:

- Early menopause – it is unusual to have a fractured hip until at least 10 years after your last period.
- Long-term steroid medicines.
- Removal of the ovaries, usually with a hysterectomy.
- Anorexia nervosa or other reasons for severe malnutrition in the past or more recently.
- Intolerance of dairy products, causing a lack of calcium.
- Some cancers.

Immediate Symptoms
You know what has happened straight away – you cannot stand up, and there is a pain in your hip. Although this can be very severe, in some cases it is surprisingly mild. One oddity: your leg turns outwards after a break.

Treatment
This always involves admission to hospital, usually for about 10 days, and surgery. The operation that causes the least complications is total hip replacement, such as so many of us have these days for bad arthritis. Exercises and physiotherapy are essential to get you back on your feet – starting on the day after the surgery.

Long-term Results
Your main problems will be continuing pain, and difficulty in becoming fully mobile again. Pain-killers and HRT beat the first problem, in the end, while determination and persistence with the exercise are essential in overcoming the second. There are also a few people who die within a

year of breaking a hip – they are likely to be particularly old or to have other diseases.

Case Study
Julie broke her hip trying to get off a train that had started to move. She was 65, and as she already had some arthritic aching and stiffness in her joints she was given a hip replacement. She made a normal recovery, but a normal convalescence did not prove as easy. Julie's big problems were:

1. Pain
2. Tiredness.

She also had difficulty with several everyday activities:
● Going up and down stairs – down was the worst
● Getting on and off buses and trains, and in and out of cars and cabs
● Housework, especially using the vacuum cleaner
● Shopping
● Lifting, carrying and bending
● Driving – though she overcame this one in five weeks.

Colles Fracture of the Wrist

This is the third of the fractures common after the menopause. It is caused by falling onto your outstretched hand, and is often the most painful.

Effects
A fractured wrist results in pain, tenderness and swelling, a limitation of movement – and the wrist looks an odd shape.

Treatment
Treatment aims at reducing the fracture – that is, getting the bones back into proper alignment, then encasing the wrist in plaster of Paris for four to six weeks.

Shoulder Fracture

This occurs less often than the other three types of fracture, but is caused by the same kind of accident as a Colles fracture. In this case the break is in the upper part of the humerus, the large bone running from elbow to shoulder. Usually it only requires immobilizing for three or four weeks, and some physiotherapy. Occasionally surgery is necessary.

Diagnostic Helpers in Osteoporosis

- Standard X-ray examination, showing the outlines of the bones and any fractures.
- QCT – Quantitative CT (computerized tomography): a scan which assesses how much bone substance has been lost. Particularly useful in checking the spine.
- DEXA (dual energy X-ray absorptiometry): a most sophisticated technique which also measures the strength of the bones in terms of calcium and other important materials. It can be applied to any bone in the body.
- Ultrasound scanning – this is very useful for assessing osteoporosis in the neck.

Treatment in Osteoporosis

HRT (Hormone Replacement Therapy)
This is the top treatment for all menopausal illness, including osteoporosis. You can go on taking it indefinitely, although after 8 to 10 years there is a slightly increased risk of breast cancer. There are sometimes side-effects such as nausea and vomiting, but these are troublesome rather than dangerous. There are also a few conditions in which you cannot take HRT (see page 56).

SERMS (Selective (o)Estrogen Receptor Modulators)
Only one type of these, raloxifene (brand name Evista), is available at present. It is recommended especially for women past the menopause who have vulnerable vertebrae and are at risk of pain and deformity in the back.

Calcitonin
This is usually taken as salmon calcitonin (salcatonin) and is particularly useful for those who cannot take HRT. It has to be taken in a nasal spray or by injection.

Other hormones that are sometimes used in osteoporosis include tamoxifen, progesterone, growth hormone and some anabolic hormones.

Non-hormonal Drugs Used in Osteoporosis
Bisphosphonates
These are the most important. They slow down the rate of bone turnover, especially by interrupting resorption (the breaking-down process). In the correct dosage, bisphosphonates encourage bones to take up calcium. Alendronate (Fosamax) is the most effective of these drugs. You take it

once a day on an empty stomach, on waking, with a full glass of water, then wait for an hour before swallowing anything else.

Calcium
This is the first-line preventative and treatment for osteoporosis, and is quicker than anything else in reducing the risk of a fracture. It interacts with several common medicines, including steroids, iron, digoxin and tetracycline, so always check with your doctor first before starting a regime of taking calcium tablets.

Hydroxyapatite (Ossopan)
Hydroxyapatite provides calcium and phosphates and has no side-effects. It is derived from bone.

Occasionally, fluoride or thiazide water tablets are also used in the treatment of osteoporosis.

Chapter 8

Heart and Artery Disease

There are two major traps laid by the menopause. Osteoporosis is one, but you can reduce the risk by rearranging your lifestyle, or ameliorate the disease with treatment. It can damage the quality of your life, but is not immediately life-threatening.

Heart and artery – cardiovascular – disease is the other big danger, and it is a definite killer of women after the menopause. It accounts for four times as many deaths as cancers of the womb, cervix and breast put together, and half of all the deaths of women. The basic cause and the reason it strikes after the change is the fall-off in sex hormones, oestrogen in particular, when the ovaries stop regularly producing eggs. All the time we have plenty of oestrogen, we women are protected from the cardiovascular disasters – coronary artery heart attack, high blood pressure and stroke – which threaten our menfolk from their late forties onwards. During the perimenopause, when the ovaries become gradually less active, we become more vulnerable to these disorders, and 8 to 10 years after our last period, the risks of cardiovascular disease are even between the sexes.

We cannot avoid having the change, but we can minimize the risks by taking sensible precautions in good time and zapping any warning symptoms if they occur.

The villain of the piece, underlying all the dangers to the cardiovascular system, is *atheroma*. *Athero* is Greek for 'porridge', and *oma* means 'a lump'. The combination refers to porridgy lumps of fatty material which form in the lining of the arteries. Atherosclerosis is the result of accumulating atheroma, so that the arteries are increasingly blocked up. This can cause trouble in several ways.

Ischaemic Heart Disease (IHD)

This is the biggest killer in the Western world. It means that not enough blood can get through the narrowed passageways of the arteries supplying the heart muscle. These are the coronary arteries, and when they are silted up you have coronary artery disease (CHD), which is only a more exact way of describing IHD.

The basic problem is the fatty gunge inside the arteries. The fat involved is *cholesterol*.

This is not as straightforward as it sounds. There are several types of cholesterol and they fall into two main groups: High-Density Lipoprotein cholesterols (HDL) and Low-Density Lipoprotein cholesterols (LDL). Oestrogen – and to a lesser extent, progesterone – control the proportions of these fats in the blood, so that HDLs in women before the change run at a higher level in relation to LDLs and to the total cholesterol level than they do in men. HDLs are kinder to the arteries than LDLs.

In general, the more the total cholesterol level, the greater the risk of CHD and the other cardiovascular disorders. For instance, if you have a total cholesterol reading of 300 mg/dl, you stand five times more chance of a heart attack (in fact, a 90% risk) than if the level is 150 mg/dl. However, there is still a substantial risk – 20% – even at the lower figure. At under 150 mg/dl of cholesterol, you are very unlikely to develop atherosclerosis – in common with the poor in Asia, Africa and Latin America. What makes life so dangerous for us is the Western style of fast living and fast food.

Risk Factors for Coronary Heart Disease and Heart Attack

- Waist-to-hip measurements in a ratio of more than 5:4
- Family members who have had cardiovascular problems before the age of 55
- Total cholesterol level in the blood of more than 150 mg/dl
- LDL more than 140 mg/dl, HDL less than 45 mg/dl
- Triglycerides (another form of fat) more than 80 mg/dl
- Diabetes, usually the middle-aged, overweight type (known as Type 2 Diabetes)
- Blood glucose (sugar) level more than 100 mg/dl
- Insulin resistance
- Increased clotting factor

These are the items you may see in a pathological report, which give you information about whether you need to cut down your fats, your sugar or your weight.

Some Factors Which Contribute to the Risk of Heart Attack or Stroke

The Downside of Oestrogen
In the form of HRT, this is the most popular treatment for CHD after the change, but it is a double-edged sword. It always reduces the tendency to atheroma, but in large doses increases the likelihood of a heart attack. This

is because it increases the risk of clotting of the blood. HRT is not a substitute for cholesterol-lowering treatment with diet and medication. Only 1 in 10 women taking HRT shows any reduction in the damaging LDL cholesterol.

The benefits of taking oestrogen in reasonable doses include an antioxidant effect, maintaining the health of the arteries; control of the proportions of HDL and LDL, stabilizing the effects of adrenalin on the heart, dilating the coronary arteries, and inhibiting the clotting mechanism.

High Blood Pressure
In the West we take it for granted that blood pressure always increases with age, but in fact it only does so among people who use an excess of salt. In the US and UK we consume 20 times as much salt as we need, much of it hidden in processed foods. Adding this to the tendency to postmenopausal atherosclerosis and overweight, it is no surprise that high blood pressure is common. Fifty percent of British and American women after the change have a blood pressure of 140/90 or more – now considered to be high.

To avoid ill-effects on your heart, the modern recommendation is to keep your blood pressure below 130/85, much lower than previously accepted. It used to be thought healthy and natural for your blood pressure to go up as you grew older. We know now that this is not the case, and that elderly people are actually more vulnerable than youngsters to high blood pressure. Their blood vessels are more fragile.

Smoking
This is not particularly associated with the menopause, but it is an important risk factor for IHD, stroke and high blood pressure. It was not until after the Second World War that women smoked on a large scale. By the 1960s they were beginning to suffer from more heart and artery diseases and also lung cancer. In 1987, lung cancer overtook breast cancer as the most lethal cancer for women, as it had been for men for some years.

Women, more often than men, go for low-yield, 'mild' cigarettes, but these are associated with just as much death and ill-health from heart disease as high-tar, high-nicotine tobacco. The risk of a heart attack is doubled for a woman after the change, if she smokes even up to 10 cigarettes a day, and there is more than 7 times the danger if she smokes 30. The only safe course is to quit. The extra risk to your heart is wiped out within a year of giving up.

Blood Sugar
Even if your blood sugar is within the normal range but is near the upper

limit, you run an increased risk of a cardiovascular problem, usually through developing diabetes. Most people with diabetes will ultimately die of a heart attack or stroke, and it raises the risk enormously for menopausal women. Cut down on sweet foods if your sugar level is approaching 10 mmol per litre.

Overweight
It seems unfair, but if you are overweight, the particular fats that cause atherosclerosis increase, and HDL, the protective type, decreases. Your blood sugar, blood pressure and insulin resistance go up – all bad news for your heart, which has to work harder and reacts by enlarging.

Stress
You run twice the risk of a heart attack after the menopause if you are consistently under stress. Check if you are in danger:

- Do people say you are bossy? This means that you take onto yourself responsibility for everyone else's behaviour, and feel you must direct and correct them.
- Are you always pressed for time?
- Do you eat your meals quickly, perhaps at your desk, instead of making them a break in which to unwind?
- Do you feel you must excel and be the best at whatever you are involved in – work, sport, sex..?
- Do you miss out on regular holidays, looking for any excuse not to down tools?
- Do you find your job unsatisfying and frustrating?
- Is your boss or partner insensitive, in your view?
- Do you have children, a demanding job and a home to run?
- Is your partner less ambitious, less focused than you, someone you can love but not look up to?

Three 'yes' answers mean you need to insert more breaks, more relaxation, more plain fun into your life.

A Sedentary Lifestyle
This danger to your cardiovascular system creeps up on you. Every new invention and 'improvement' is aimed at preventing you from moving a muscle, except to press a button. It would be inconceivable, today, to choose to walk 15 miles to hear a sermon, as Charles Wesley often did, or, like Dr Johnson, to cover the same distance on foot to clear his brain. And if we do take any exercise we are apt to expect pounds to fall away. You need to walk a mile to use up 100 calories, the equivalent of one sweet biscuit; 6

miles for a Big Mac; and 35 miles to burn off a single pound (2.2 kg).

However, it is worthwhile to exercise regularly. A 2-mile walk daily or 40 minutes' brisk exercise three times a week is enough to reduce the risk of a heart attack by more than 30% – after a year. Then you must keep it up. The cheering news is that there seems to be no extra risk to your heart from drinking coffee, shortage of sleep, marital status or where you live.

Case Study
Janet totted up her personal risk factors for a heart attack when her brother, three years her senior at 53, had his bypass operation. He had already been through two heart attacks and his doctor did not want him to risk a third. Janet was now in the perimenopause and had not had a period for two months. Her brother's illness indicated that she had a hereditary tendency to atheroma – this was the first risk factor, apart from the menopause itself. She also knew that she could do with losing three or four pounds. She had put on a little weight when she gave up smoking, but it was better to have kicked that habit than to have achieved her ideal weight. Her doctor agreed, but took her blood pressure as a check.

At 145/92 it was high but not dangerously so, and reducing her weight, a matter of diet, might improve her blood pressure without the need for medication. The doctor suggested that it would be beneficial to cut out refined white sugar and refined white bread, cakes and biscuits – making it up with more vegetables, fruit and wholegrain cereals. Saturated fats – in meat, butter, cream, processed foods and pre-packaged dishes – should not exceed 10 g, and dietary cholesterol not more than 300 mg daily. Achieving these levels meant Janet had to study the small-print nutritional information on her foods.

Finally, there was stress, which could also be relevant. Janet was PA to the manager of a large motor firm. Sales were down and he took his anxieties out on Janet, finding fault with whatever she did.

For the rest, she was active but did not take any exercise; her blood sugar and cholesterol levels were well within normal limits, and her one son was no problem now – an adult, living with his girlfriend. Janet's own divorce was history and she had come to enjoy the freedom it gave her. In line with the idea that it was ineffective to try shutting the stable door after the horse had gone, Janet decided to take preventative steps against coronary disease straight away – before it had a chance to develop. She tightened up the slack in her life with more exercise, less sweet and fatty food, new interests – swimming and local history – and, when the opportunity arose, a change of job. She is now in administration instead of being at the mercy of the moods of one boss.

At the last count, Janet's blood pressure was 128/80, a safe level, and her weight a respectable 8 st 9 lbs for her height of 5 ft 1 (54 kg, 1.56 m). She is currently working on cultivating a more easygoing outlook, something her colleagues appreciate.

How Heart and Artery Problems Show Themselves

There are two important indicators that your heart and arteries are under strain:
- High blood pressure: it usually causes no symptoms in itself but is quickly discovered in any medical check.
- Shortness of breath, so that you find you cannot walk and talk at the same time, especially uphill, or you get puffed hurrying for a bus.

Transient Ischaemic Attack (TIA)

This is a short-lived reduction in the blood supply to the heart or brain, due to one or more of the narrowed arteries of atherosclerosis becoming blocked by the formation of a clot, kinking of a blood vessel when you hold your neck at a particular angle, or simple muscle spasm in the wall of an artery. The effects may last for a few minutes only, or as long as 24 hours.

The symptoms depend on which blood vessels are put out of service, temporarily. You may have vertigo, lose your sense of balance so that you cannot walk safely, feel faint or see double, or a hand or limb may feel numb or weak. A TIA warns you of the danger of a stroke, but since it is, by definition, transient, treatment of the episode is not as important as overall care of your cardiovascular system, with, for example, control of your blood pressure.

Angina

Angina – a chest pain that feels like a tight band or cramp in the heart muscle – is another way your heart may signal that it is in difficulty.

Common Triggers of an Angina Attack
- Taking a walk in an icy wind
- A heavy meal
- Overexertion, for instance lifting something very weighty
- Strong emotion – from terror to happy excitement
- Dwelling on negative thoughts such as some kind of personal disaster
- An increased level of the thyroid hormone, thyroxine, which makes your heart beat too fast. Paradoxically, a severe shortage of thyroxine, as in those suffering myxoedema, also affects the heart by worsening atherosclerosis.

49

- Lying flat – called *decubitus angina*. In this position your heart is at a disadvantage for pumping – it works more comfortably if you are sitting up.

The underlying risk factors are the same as those which apply to IHD.

Coronary Heart Attack (also called Myocardial Ischaemia)

Sometimes a heart attack strikes out of the blue – you are just getting out of your car – or you may have felt unduly tired over several days beforehand, without knowing why. The central symptom is pain – it has been likened to red-hot wires twisting in your chest, or like very severe angina. Unlike angina, the pain is not dispersed by GTN (glycerol trinitrate) tablets and you enter a state of shock – becoming pale, sweaty and acutely anxious. You may vomit, and you feel faint because your blood pressure falls. This means your heart has to beat faster, but your pulse is weak.

Treatment will start with an injection to ease the pain, and from then on you will be given various medicines, and possibly surgery later on. Rehabilitation – building up to a good level of health, perhaps as good as it had been before – takes weeks. It is time to review your lifestyle and the risks to your cardiovascular system: diet, habits, exercise, stress and weight.

Stroke

The name conjures up what usually happens: it is like a sudden blow, knocking the victim unconscious. Less commonly there is what is called an 'evolving stroke' in which the symptoms emerge over a few days. The medical name for a stroke, cardiovascular accident, is also explanatory. A blood vessel to part of the brain may get blocked by a clot or a fragment of atheroma lodging in it. Less often, a tiny vessel, weakened by atherosclerosis and high blood pressure, may break down and bleed. Either way, some tissue is damaged.

The signs vary, and may start with a coma, but often include paralysis of an arm or a leg on one side, and sometimes loss of sensation. Speech may be jumbled, so that the wrong words come out. Recovery can go on for as long as a year, with excellent results, so persistent rehabilitation treatment is essential, but there is always a danger of further strokes.

Chapter 9

Hormone Replacement Therapy: Why Should You Take It?

Back in 1889, a 72-year-old French doctor, Charles Brown-Sequard, was desperate to regain his youthful sexual vigour. His was the first attempt at hormone replacement therapy, giving himself injections of ground-up dogs' testicles, blood and semen. After the first three doses he felt wonderfully rejuvenated and the patent medicine manufacturers jumped on the band wagon – but sadly, it all came to nothing. It had been a mammoth placebo response – a temporary phenomenon due to hope and faith.

The true account of the development of hormone replacement treatment, which has, indeed, been described as 'the elixir of eternal youth', is a woman's story. It began with baseball and two young men in the same faculty team at Washington University, St Louis, Missouri. Edgar Allen, a zoologist, and Edward Doisy, a biochemist, palled up and compared notes about their work, finally combining their skills to find a female sex hormone in pigs' ovaries. In 1929 they isolated *oestrone*, one of the family of oestrogens. By 1933, two others had been discovered: *oestriol* and *oestradiol*.

The hunt was on. The very next year another, different type of sex hormone, *progesterone*, was found in the empty follicle when an ovum, or egg, had been released from it. This event is of course called ovulation, and occurs regularly during a woman's reproductive years.

Oestrogen Manufacture

This takes place in the follicles of the ovaries, little blister-like structures containing fluid, in each of which an ovum may develop and mature before release at the rate of one a month The ingredients for the hormone are cholesterol and acetate.

Progesterone Production

This follows after ovulation. While oestrogen stimulates growth and activity, progesterone inhibits it. There is a changing interplay between the two hormones. Oestrogen peaks at ovulation, around the 14th day of the menstrual cycle, and hits its lowest point a week later, Day 21. Progesterone predominates then, but declines by the end of the cycle.

Sex hormone production ticks over at a low level until age 9 or 10, when the breast buds are like little pimples on the girl's chest. From then on it increases rapidly, reaching its all-time high during pregnancy. It begins to falter from age 35 to 40. This is reflected in the advice to young women to have their first child, at least, before reaching 35, and in the huge numbers now seeking fertility treatment because they have left it too late. The current trend is to spend the most fertile years building up a career or in other ways consolidating one's place in life.

HRT Comes into Use

As far back as the 1940s, doctors were treating women with oestrogen if their ovaries were not functioning or had been removed – straight hormone replacement therapy. An Englishman, Dr Robert Wilson, motivated by sympathy for the sufferings of his mother during her menopause, moved to the States to devote the rest of his life to researching and explaining the benefits of HRT. His book, *Feminine Forever*, came out in 1966. Joan Jenkins, founder of the Women's Health Concern Centre in 1972, remains an ardent disciple of Dr Wilson and has taken HRT for 30 years.

It was in the late 1960s that HRT came into general use for those with menopausal symptoms – a natural follow-on from the contraceptive pill, which was also based on oestrogen. For the first time there was a treatment which relieved the misery of hot flushes and night sweats in particular, which had made the change something to be dreaded. The effects seemed almost magical, and HRT grew rapidly in popularity. Until, that is, 1970.

Case Study
Julia, turned 50 in 1970, was one of a new breed of businesswomen who prided themselves on being able to meet and beat any man on equal terms. She found it particularly galling when she began having terrific hot flushes, during which her face would go lobster red and sweaty. She also suffered badly from night sweats and disrupted sleep. Julia had been one of the first in her set to go on the contraceptive pill, and she did not hesitate now to follow her doctor's suggestion of taking HRT.

It was precisely then that the cancer panic broke out. A definite link had emerged between HRT and cancer of the womb, and there were fears that there was an increased risk of breast cancer. Julia was alarmed, especially as her mother had developed breast cancer in her seventies. She gave up HRT, causing an unpleasant rebound of her symptoms, but found relief from some herbal remedies including Agnus Castus and Black Haw. A few years later, with the use of progesterone, the scare about cancer of the womb abated, but still Julia worried about breast cancer.

The problem was that the oestrogen, which was effectual for the menopausal symptoms, also stimulated the lining of the womb to go on growing, with a high risk of malignancy developing. Without ovulation there were neither periods nor progesterone to check it. Once this was realized, the answer was clear: progesterone or one of its analogues has been given to every woman taking oestrogen for menopausal symptoms, except those who have had a hysterectomy. The progestogen is given during the latter part of what would have been the menstrual cycle, or continuously with the oestrogen. This is the modern style of HRT. The danger of cancer of the womb is no higher with HRT than without.

Several big surveys on the incidence of breast cancer in women taking HRT have shown that it does not increase the risk of breast cancer, even in those who have had the disease previously. Nevertheless, there remain some sceptics, and it seems prudent to avoid HRT if you have a strong history of breast cancer in the family, or have had it yourself and recovered.

How HRT May Help You

Not only is HRT the best, and to all intents and purposes the only effective treatment for the vasomotor symptoms of the menopause, it is in the forefront of prevention. It offers considerable protection against osteoporosis and heart and artery disease in the postmenopause, and there is good evidence that it also reduces the risk of Alzheimer's disease and colon cancer – both apparently unconnected with the reproductive system.

In essence, HRT compensates for the drastic fall-off in oestrogen production by the ovaries when you stop ovulating. This leaves you with a third to a half of the previous amount, as measured in the blood plasma. It is a matter of urgency for those who have had a premature menopause, for whatever reason, including surgery, to replace some of their loss. Without this they are likely to have exceptionally severe symptoms and suffer serious damage to their bones and cardiovascular system.

The Benefits of HRT

- Dramatic alleviation of hot flushes, night sweats and palpitations
- Reversal of the uncomfortable dryness of the vagina, which affects intercourse and impairs your sex life
- Improves incontinence of urine, both the stress and the urge types
- Ameliorates symptoms in the urogenital area: burning and itching when you pass water, frequency and a tendency to episodes of cystitis – inflammation of the bladder
- Slight reduction in the propensity to put on weight, especially in the abdomen, thighs and hips – contrary to what many women believe

- Evidence of some protection against Alzheimer's disease, colon cancer (but not cancer of the rectum), and possibly Parkinson's disease. There is three times the risk of this last disease in women who have had a hysterectomy, but this is reduced if they are on HRT.
- Reduction in periodontal (round the teeth) disease and tooth loss
- Improvement in psychological symptoms such as depression, lack of energy and anxiety. Eighty percent of women taking HRT feel more in control of their lives and more positive about their future.
- Boost to your sexual interest and enjoyment. In a recent research study by the Royal College of Physicians, more than 50% of menopausal women said that, since starting on HRT, they thought about sex more often than they had 10 years ago. Some had noticed their interest declining since their 30s, while 82% of menopausal women who were taking HRT said they enjoyed intercourse more than previously, compared with 69% of those not on the hormone treatment.

Case Study

Marion worried about losing her husband. At 49 she was slightly too plump, but felt hideously fat, old and unattractive. Because she was depressed she had little energy and did not bother to look after herself apart from a little comfort eating. This only made matters worse and made her feel guilty. She was resigned to a failing marriage, middle age and a downhill progression to a lonely old age. No wonder she slept badly. She consulted her GP about the insomnia. He noticed her lack-lustre appearance and downbeat attitude, and asked her about her periods. They were dwindling, which made her feel less feminine than ever.

Although Marion did not have the classic symptoms of the menopause, her doctor suggested HRT rather than an antidepressant. To her surprise, after about six weeks she felt as though she were coming to life. Her mood lifted, her interest in things revived, her energy increased, and she took her weight problem in hand. Most significantly, the sexual side of the marriage was revitalized. Her husband appreciated this, especially as he had just discovered Viagra. Their relationship developed a new lease of life.

The advent of the menopause, a definite milestone in maturity, may nudge us into thinking about our bodies and the future. The years 50-60-70 are usually good years healthwise if you have a reasonable lifestyle and are not overweight. Statistically most women sail through these years unless they are excessively overweight or unlucky. There are two spectres that can haunt us when we contemplate the long term – cancer and Alzheimer's disease. HRT is good news on both counts.

Cancer of the Colon
This is the third most common cancer in women, and commonly crops up between the ages of 50 and 60. There are reports that it is less likely to do so if you are taking HRT or have done recently.

Breast Cancer
This is always an emotive subject as a top cause of death from cancer in women. It is often the centre of controversy. Does oestrogen treatment increase the risks or reduce them? The major risk factors are:
- Your genes, particularly if your mother had the illness
- Your age – breast cancer does not peak at a particular age, but occurs more frequently as you grow older
- Having your children late and starting your periods early
- Previous harmless breast lumps
- Drinking and smoking
- Overweight
- Using the contraceptive pill – a very slight effect
- HRT: in the first 10 years of taking HRT, the benefits far outweigh any risk. After 10 years on HRT the odds shorten from 22 to 1 to 20 to 1 against developing breast cancer, and after 15 years it is 17 to 1 against.

You can weigh up the risk for yourself. In several research surveys there appeared to be no extra risk from taking HRT. Screening by self-examination, your doctor's check and a mammogram are useful precautions.

Alzheimer's Disease
This includes what we used to call 'senile dementia'. It comprises a fall-off in general sharpness and memory in particular, and is closely linked with age. Since we are all living longer in the 21st century, there is a longer period when we are at risk and we hear of more sufferers. While 3% of women between 65 and 74 are likely to develop the illness, the proportion increases to 47% at 85, and 50% from 95 onwards.

Some researchers have found that the risk is halved in women who have been taking HRT for a year or more, or who have stopped it only recently. The theory is that oestrogen improves the blood flow to the brain, stimulates the brain cells and increases levels of one of the chemical messengers, acetylcholine. Oestrogen is also an antioxidant, which has the effect of slowing down the ageing process in the tissues. There is hopeful evidence that HRT helps to prevent Alzheimer's disease, or at least delays its onset, and after that reduces the symptoms, especially the poor memory.

With such tremendous potential benefits, it is not surprising that two major authorities strongly advocate the use of HRT: The European Consensus Conference on the Menopause, which stated in its report of 1996 that most menopausal women should take HRT, and The United States Preventive Services Task Force, which advised, also in 1996, that all women of menopausal age should be counselled on the value of the treatment. It also says something that 80% of women in the change in the US and Canada are on HRT, while the UK lags behind with a 20-30% uptake. The exceptions in Britain are women doctors and gynaecologists and doctors' wives – who are more than twice as likely to take HRT. Presumably these groups are better informed than other people. However, neither of the main reports, nor even Dr Wilson, whose mission in life was to promote HRT, suggests that it is suitable or even safe for every woman.

Case Study
Greta was 52. She had four children, spaced out over 12 years – the youngest was now 10. Greta noticed that she had been putting on weight lately. She enjoyed her food and had a sweet tooth, so she did not think anything of it until her period did not come on the expected date. She had relaxed over contraception because she felt there was very little risk of her getting pregnant. She and her husband did not have sex all that often these days.

Then she began to have doubts – the period was not just late, it did not arrive at all. Could she possibly be pregnant? She warmed to the idea, and became convinced that was the cause of the missing period. It was around this time that the palpitations began, and waves of faintness and cold sweat swept over her. The doctor checked her urine and told her that she was not pregnant, while a hormone test on her blood showed that she was in the menopause. Greta's symptoms were relieved soon after she started on HRT. This would have been dangerous to the embryo had she been pregnant, so the doctor's tests were a necessary precaution.

You Must NOT Take HRT If:
- You could be pregnant
- You have cancer of the breast or the womb – cancers of the ovary or the cervix are not risk factors
- You suffer from acute liver disease – hepatitis A, B or C or cirrhosis, with abnormal liver function tests
- There is unexplained bleeding from the vagina, which might be due to cancer of the womb
- You have venous thrombosis – clotting in a vein – and embolism when a fragment of clot lodges in an artery
- You have endometriosis – a disorder of the lining of the womb

- You suffer from otosclerosis: in this form of deafness HRT may cause a permanent deterioration

Other Reasons for Your Doctor to Advise You Against HRT
- Family members with breast cancer
- Fibroids: these are harmless tumours in the muscle of the uterus, but they are sensitive to oestrogen and may bleed heavily and cause swelling of the abdomen with HRT. The good news is that fibroids shrink as the natural oestrogen supply diminishes in the change, so are unlikely to cause trouble. If you have had a hysterectomy for fibroids or any other cause, there is no reason not to take HRT.
- Gallstones currently or in the past: steroid molecules from the oestrogen of HRT are taken into the gall bladder and increase the likelihood of stone formation. There is no risk if you have had a cholecystectomy – removal of the gall bladder.
- Several relatives who have had thromboses or embolism
- Breast lumps which are not cancerous – there is an increased risk of a cancer developing – but only if you continue with HRT for 10 years or more
- Obesity – not just plumpness
- Migraine headaches
- Multiple sclerosis – you need to find out by trial and error whether HRT improves the symptoms or worsens them.
- Epilepsy: theoretically, extra oestrogen may trigger a fit, but progesterone, the other hormone given in HRT, has the reverse effect.

Special care and monitoring is needed if you have high blood pressure, diabetes or severe varicose veins.

Urgent Reasons to Stop Taking HRT
- Migraine-type headache – that is, involving disturbances in your vision, nausea and perhaps vomiting, and the headache tends to be on one side only
- Repeated severe headaches of any type
- Visual disturbances coming out of the blue
- Jaundice
- Sudden breathlessness
- Signs of blood clotting

Other reasons for giving up HRT are severe side-effects or incompatibility with medication you have to take for another condition. These are considered in Chapter 10.

Chapter 10

Hormone Replacement Therapy: How to Take It

The contraceptive pill caused a revolution in women's sex lives, and HRT, using the same components, made an equally dramatic breakthrough for those of us facing the menopause – with its inconvenient, often embarrassing symptoms and its serious long-term health risks. The basic ingredients are the female sex hormones: oestrogens and progestogens.

Oestrogens

Our own bodies and those of some animals produce three types of oestrogen: oestrone, oestradiol and oestriol. There is also a range of synthetic oestrogens. The natural (non-synthetic) oestrogens used in HRT are prepared from horse's urine. The name of one of the best-known HRT tablets, Premarin, is a give-away: *Pre* from pregnant, *mar* from mare and *in* from urine. It is these natural oestrogens that are mainly used in HRT.

Synthetic hormones are man-made and similar chemically to our own oestrogens, but more powerful. Ethinyloestradiol is the one that crops up most frequently, in many different contraceptive pills including the 'morning after' pill, Schering PC4. Mestranol and dienoestrol are other synthetic oestrogens. They are used in oral contraceptives where a stronger effect is required than with HRT, which aims not to interfere with nature but only to compensate mildly for the shortfall in oestrogen.

Another group of 'natural' oestrogens are the phyto-oestrogens. These are substances derived from plants which have some of the properties of oestrogens but do not resemble them chemically and do not have all the same effects. Well-known oestrogenic plants are Ginseng, Evening Primrose and Elder. They are not used in HRT, but are given in the menopause by some alternative therapists.

Progestogens

The other group of female hormones, the progestogens, counteract and balance the effects of oestrogen. This is especially important in preventing the overgrowth of the endometrium (the lining of the womb), when a woman is given extra oestrogen to replace partly what is lacking as ovulation tapers off. The usual make-up of HRT combines a natural oestrogen with a synthetic progestogen. This is because the only natural progestogen manufactured in the body is progesterone, which is ineffective if you take it by mouth. What little is absorbed is rapidly destroyed in the digestive system, so synthetic products must be used in hormone replacement. Those in common use are norethisterone, levonorgestrel and gestodene.

Androgens

These male hormones, of which testosterone is the best known, are increasingly prescribed for women in the menopause, especially in North America, together with oestrogen and a progestogen. They are normally produced in small quantities by the ovaries and are concerned with sexual drive. Their production diminishes together with that of oestrogen at the menopause. Some menopausal symptoms, for example loss of libido – sexual interest – lack of physical energy and headaches, may be improved by an androgen such as methyltestosterone. Like progesterone, ordinary testosterone is poorly absorbed by mouth: injections or implants are more effective.

HRT is available in a variety of forms – from tablets to suppositories to gels – each designed for a particular situation. For most people, however, tablets taken by mouth are the most convenient way of taking the medication. There are no dietary restrictions, nor does it matter when you take them. HRT doesn't make you drowsy, nor does it create a dependency, however long you are on it. Alcohol does not interact with HRT, and there are very few other medicines except anti-clotting drugs like Warfarin, taken by mouth, which become less effective as a result. Heparin, however, given by injection, is unaffected. Smoking is just as damaging to the heart and arteries if you are on HRT, although HRT reduces the risk of coronary heart disease in a non-smoker.

Taking the Tablets

First of all your doctor must check you over, including taking your blood pressure and running blood tests, to make sure that HRT is safe and suitable for you. That done, the first problem is when you should take it.

When Should You Start HRT?

If you are plagued by vasomotor symptoms – flushes, sweats, palpitations or dryness of the vagina – as soon as possible. You will be eager to benefit from the relief afforded, in most cases, by HRT. It takes about 7 to 10 days to kick in. The other main reason for taking HRT is to protect your bones from osteoporosis and your heart from coronary artery disease. You have to take the tablets for three or four months before they have an effect in these areas.

Not every woman suffers from the specific symptoms of the menopause, and you may not feel you want to bother with medication just yet. Your ovaries will continue to make a certain amount of oestrogen for several years after your periods have stopped, and this may be enough to keep the symptoms at bay. However, your oestrogen level will have started falling steadily two or three years before your last period, and your bones, arteries and less vital organs, such as your skin, will feel the lack. The least you can do is to supply your bones with extra calcium in the form of dairy produce or supplements, and a daily capsule of fish liver oil to provide the vitamin D needed to help you absorb it.

An Added Complication
If you have been taking an oral contraceptive which induces regular bleeds, you will not be able to tell when your ovaries are no longer able to provide the hormones that cause normal periods.

On your 50th birthday, or thereabouts, it is time to change to a barrier type of contraception – cap or condom – so that you can assess whether you are in your perimenopause or the menopause itself. For maximum benefit you need not wait until then but start on HRT as soon as your ovaries signal that they are retiring. They do this by a change in your periods, or the advent of menopausal symptoms.

How Long Should You Stay on HRT?

Three to five years is usually long enough on HRT to see off any troublesome symptoms, and many women give it up after about 18 months. However, there is no upper limit healthwise, and indeed the longer you continue the better for your bones, joints, heart and arteries. Joan Jenkins, Robert Wilson's follower, flourished on HRT for 30 years. Oddly enough, it is those who are young and trendy by nature who tend to remain on HRT throughout their 60s. They benefit both physically and psychologically, delaying the ageing process – but the price is the inconvenience of withdrawal bleeds for a longer time.

There is a small but progressive disadvantage in continuing the tablets for more than 10 years – the risks of breast and womb cancer increase slightly.

Different Types of Tablet

1. Oestrogen-only HRT
2. 'Sequential combined' HRT, incorporating an oestrogen and
    a progestogen in one pack
3. 'No bleed HRT' or 'Continuous combined HRT'

Oestrogen-only Tablets

These are for you only if you have had a hysterectomy, but it makes no difference to your choice of medication whether or not your ovaries have
been removed (oophorectomy). If you still have a womb, taking oestrogen
alone now that you are producing much less progesterone increases the
risk by 50% of your developing a cancer of the womb lining – endometrium – and, to a lesser extent, that of breast cancer.

Most of the oestrogen-only tablets contain oestradiol: the exceptions are
Premarin and Harmonin, which comprise a mix of the natural oestrogens,
and Harmogen, containing oestrone, and Ovestin, which contains oestriol
only.

Brand name	Oestrogen	Dosage
Climaval	oestradiol	1mg, 2mg
Elleste solo	oestradiol	1mg, 2mg
Progynova	oestradiol	1mg, 2mg
Zumenon	oestradiol	1mg, 2 mg
Harmonin	mixture	0.27mg, 0.6mg, 1.4mg
Premarin	mixture	0.625mg, 1.25mg, 2.5mg
Harmogen	oestrone	0.93mg
Ovestin	oestriol	1mg

The dosage depends partly on your response to the medication – for
instance whether you have any side-effects, and partly on your main reason for taking HRT -

● to relieve menopausal symptoms, especially hot flushes, sweats and
    dry vagina
● to protect you against osteoporosis and coronary heart disease.

Controlling symptoms requires a higher dose than avoiding symptoms
you have not got (prophylaxis).

'Sequential Combined' Oestrogen/Progestogen Tablets

Most of us have not had a hysterectomy when we are considering HRT. In that case, when you take oestrogen it is essential also to take progestogen for 10-14 days in every month. Calendar packs contain tablets in fixed doses of both oestrogen and progestogen tablets, and all you need do is take them in order. Sometimes your doctor will want to vary the type or dose of either one of the hormones, and this may be achieved with separate oestrogen-only and progestogen tablets. This is most likely if you are having troublesome side-effects or if you are a heavy smoker. In the latter case you may need a bigger dose of oestrogen because tobacco accelerates its metabolism, clearing it from your system more rapidly.

In this situation it works most conveniently if you start with the progestogen on the 1st of each month, with the oestrogen following. The bleed then comes around the middle of the month. Bleeding at any other time needs investigating.

Brand name	Oestrogen	Progestogen
Climagest	oestradiol (1mg, 2mg)	norethisterone (1mg)
Cycloprogynova	oestradiol (1mg, 2mg)	levonorgestrel (0.25mg, 0.5mg)
Elleste duet	oestradiol (1mg, 2mg)	norethisterone (1mg)
Fermoston 1/10	oestradiol (1mg)	dydrogesterone (10mg)
Fermoston 2/10	oestradiol (2mg)	dydrogesterone (10mg)
Fermoston 2/20	oestradiol (2mg)	dydrogesterone (20mg)
Trisequens	oestradiol (2mg, 2mg, 1mg or 4mg, 4mg, 1mg)	norethisterone (1mg)
Premique cycle	mixed (0.625mg)	medroxyprogesterone (10mg)
Prempak C	mixed (0.625mg, 1.25mg)	norgestrel (150mcg)
Tridestra	oestradiol (2mg)	medroxyprogesterone (20mg)

Tridestra produces a bleed every three months, instead of monthly like the other sequential combined preparations. With Tridestra you take the oestrogen continuously for 10 weeks, then add the progestogen for 2 weeks. Finally there is a seven-day gap with no medication which brings on the withdrawal bleed, and the pattern is repeated.

'No Bleed' or Continuous CombinedTablets

The big bonus of the menopause is not having periods, and it can be irksome to continue with monthly bleeds when you are on HRT. The bleeds are not, of course, periods but the withdrawal effect of automatically stopping the oestrogen component in the sequential tablets. An added snag is that if you are subject to the premenstrual syndrome it may continue to trouble you in association with these 'pseudo-periods'. Tridestra cuts the frequency down, but you cannot change to a no-bleed regime until you have not had a period for 15 months – some gynaecologists prefer you to wait for two years or until you are 54. After that you can take oestrogen and progestogen together, in one tablet, without a break, so there is no withdrawal.

Brand name	Oestrogen	Progestogen
Climesse	*oestradiol (2mg)*	*norethisterone (0.7mg)*
Elleste Duet Conti	*oestradiol (2mg)*	*norethisterone (1mg)*
Kliofem	*oestradiol (2mg)*	*norethisterone (1mg)*
Kliovance	*oestradiol (1mg)*	*norethisterone (0.5mg)*
Nuvelle continuous	*oestradiol (2mg)*	*norethisterone (1mg)*
Femoston Conti	*oestradiol (1mg)*	*dydrogesterone (5mg)*
Premique	*mixed (0.625mg)*	*medroxyprogesterone (5mg)*

Case Study

Jennifer had been a sufferer from the premenstrual syndrome, PMS, since she was 30. From the mixed bag of symptoms ascribed to it, she had mood swings with extreme irritability at times, backache, bloating with water retention, and headaches. She tried a variety of treatments, from relaxation training to progesterone suppositories, but had been disappointed, particularly when the oral contraceptive made no difference. She adjusted her diet to avoid the possibility of dips in her blood sugar.

Jennifer also consulted an alternative therapist and took vitamin B6, pyridoxine, and Evening Primrose oil for several months, but as she moved into her mid-forties the PMS got worse – a common result of the sex hormone production becoming increasingly irregular, particularly with the reduction in progesterone. When Jennifer was 48 her doctor arranged a blood test which showed that she was well into the perimenopause. She was delighted when he suggested that she should start on HRT and prescribed a sequential combined oestrogen/progestogen tablet. Jennifer had banked on HRT relieving the syndrome – but it continued as before. She gave up coffee, tea, sugar, salt and cigarettes – all the stimulants she enjoyed. The result was that fatigue was added to her bundle of symptoms.

Her gynaecologist suggested changing to a different formulation of HRT, hoping to find one that suited her – in vain. He also suggested trying out an increased dose of progestogen. This is standard treatment for PMS in the ordinary way, but it had never helped Jennifer much in the past, and now seemed to make her worse.

It seemed unbearable to think she might have to wait for several years for her menopause to come and go before she could escape from PMS, but meanwhile she found it helpful to take Tridestra. At least it cut down the number of attacks to four times a year. She also took water tablets in the week before a 'period' to combat the water retention. From her 49th birthday onwards, the PMS began gradually to lessen, and since her 50th she has had no more.

Non-hormonal Oral Tablets

There are two types of medication which act similarly to HRT although they are not strictly hormones.

SERMs (Selective (o)Estrogen Receptor Modulators)
These act by blocking the effect of oestrogen, including your own, on the breasts while not interfering with its preventative action on bone loss and heart and artery disorders. Tamoxifen is a SERM used in breast cancer, but it makes menopausal symptoms worse.

The SERM suitable for menopausal women is raloxifene (Evista). It carries no increased risk of breast or uterine cancer, as oestrogen may, but provides the same protection against osteoporosis and coronary artery disease. It raises the level of HDL (high density lipoproteins), the beneficial form of cholesterol, increases bone strength and reduces the risk of blood clots. It does not, however, help with vasomotor symptoms, and in fact flushes, sweats and palpitations may become worse. The only other possible side-effects are mild cramps in the leg and slight ankle swelling.

The dose is one 60-mg tablet daily.

Tibolone (Livial)
This is a synthetic chemical, a gonadomimetic which mimics the effect of both oestrogen and progesterone like no-bleed combined HRT. No extra progestogen is needed. It is particularly useful if you have had endometriosis at any time, since it does not stimulate the lining of the womb like oestrogen.

Tibolone relieves hot flushes and the other vasomotor symptoms, and improves a low mood or loss of interest in sex. It is also protective of the bones. There are occasionally side-effects such as ankle swelling, increased facial hair and acne, muscle aches, skin irritation or itching. This is partly due to its locking on to the testosterone receptors. If you start tibolone sooner than about 18 months after your last-of-all period, you are likely to have irregular bleeding.

HRT by Other Routes than the Mouth

Disadvantages of taking HRT by mouth are that the medication passes through the liver and a lot of the dose is lost. There is also a possibility of nausea.

Transdermal Preparations are one alternative. Transdermal just means 'through the skin'. Oestrogens and progestogens pass through the skin easily.

Patches

Patches are a convenient transdermal way of delivering oestrogen to the body. They come in two types: 'reservoir' and 'matrix' and either produces an adequate amount of oestrogen. The former is a little more inclined to cause skin problems – affecting up to 5% of users. The culprit is the alcohol needed in the reservoir type, and it helps to wave the patch in the air before attaching it.

Applying a Patch
The art is to get it to stick firmly. Choose a non-hairy place below the waist, but not at the waist because it will be exposed to a lot of rubbing there. It is important to avoid the breasts. The skin must be clean and really dry, free of sweat or of skin lotion. Wait 15 minutes after a bath or shower so that there is no moisture lurking in the folds. Press the patch firmly in place, holding it against the skin with your fingertips for a count of 20, with special care round the edges.

Most patches are changed twice a week, but a few remain in place for a week. It does no harm to have a moderately warm bath or go swimming with the patch in place, but if you intend to have a long, hot soak you can remove the patch, resting it on non-sticky plastic or foil, and re-apply it later. You can do this about three times before it loses its adhesive power.

Use a different site each time.

The oestrogen used in patches is always oestradiol, a type we make ourselves, and the dosage varies in different brands.

To be applied twice weekly:

Menorest	37.5, 50 or 75 microgams
Evorel	25, 50, 75 or 100 mcg
Dermastril	25, 50 or 100 mcg
Fematrix	40 or 80 mcg
Elleste-solo MX	40 or 80 mcg

To be applied weekly:

Femseven	50, 75 or 100 mcg
ProgynovaTS	50 mcg

For those with an intact womb using oestrogen-only patches, a progestogen must be taken for 12-14 days of each 28:

Combinations

Estrapak	8 oestradiol patches plus 12 norethisterone tablets
Evorel-pak	8 oestradiol patches plus 12 norethisterone tablets
Femapak	8 oestradiol patches plus 14 dydrogesterone tablets (all for 1 month)
Estracombi	12 oestradiol patches plus 12 oestradiol/norethisterone patches: 2 weeks on each, alternating
Evorel Conti	oestradiol/norethisterone patches given continuously, changing the patch twice a week
Evorel Sequi	oestradiol and oestradiol/norethisterone patches alternating every 2 weeks

Gels

Like patches, these provide a steady input of hormone, unlike tablets taken by mouth, and they never cause nausea. Gels are particularly popular in France, and are now available in the UK. You rub the gel into the inner sides of your arms and legs and the lower part of your body: a template of how much skin to cover is supplied with the pack. The gel must be left to dry for a few minutes, and no creams or lotions should be applied for an hour, nor must the skin be washed in that time. Gels are rather messy, but they seldom cause skin irritation or any other side-effect. One application gives about as much oestrogen as a 50-mcg patch.

Oestrogel	oestradiol 0.6%
Sandrena	oestradiol in 0.5-mg and 1-mg single doses

Vaginal Creams

These are supplied with an applicator and are inserted well into the vagina. You start with two applicator doses daily, changing after two weeks to one dose daily for a further fortnight. Then you can continue with a maintenance regime of one applicator-dose once to three times a week, depending on how comfortable your vagina has become. Vaginal creams are excellent for a dry, sore vagina – vaginitis – and are also effective against hot flushes and sweats. With prolonged use they may possibly stimulate the womb lining, with the risk of encouraging a cancerous growth. A check-up after a few months is important and you might need to take a progestogen, for instance norethisterone or dydrogesterone tablets, as with other oestrogen – only preparations. Most people do not need to use a vaginal cream continuously, but for periods of 6-8 weeks from time to time.

Ortho Dienoestrol	*dienoestrol 0.01% cream*
Ortho-gynest	*oestriol 0.01% cream*
Ovestin	*oestriol 0.1% cream*
Premarin	*mixed oestrogens 1 – 2 g daily as cream*

Other Vaginal Medication
Ortho-gynest pessary, with oestriol: insert one in the vagina in the evening, reducing to twice weekly as symptoms improve.
Reassess in three months.

Tampovagan pessary, with stilboestrol: two inserted high in the vagina at night, for two to three weeks.

Vagifem vaginal tablets, with oestradiol – one to be inserted high up in the vagina daily for two weeks, then twice a week – reassess after three months.

Estring vaginal ring, with oestradiol: this releases the hormone slowly and lasts about three months.

These preparations are mainly used for vaginal symptoms, but may also provide an alternative way of providing oestrogen. A progestogen may be needed, as with other oestrogen-only preparations.

Regular check-ups are important for anyone on long-term hormonal medication.

Implants
An implant consists of a pellet or group of pellets inserted into the fatty layer under the skin. A local anaesthetic makes this painless. In most

cases it is oestrogen that is implanted, but in a few cases testosterone is used to pep up the sexual drive, boost self-confidence and improve the mood. Progesterone implants are also made, including one with six pellets compressed into a tiny cylinder measuring 11.8 by 3.2 mm.

The oestrogen implants maintain steady levels of the hormone, and these are higher than with any other method – although within the normal premenopausal range. A progestogen must be taken at the same time, and continued for two years after the oestrogen has been stopped – rather annoyingly. Tachyphylaxis1 is a phenomenon that sometimes develops with implants. Normally the implants last for five to six months before they need renewing, but in some cases the time between inserting the implant and the return of menopausal symptoms becomes progressively shorter.

Progestogen Preparations

Suppository
Cyclogest
This provides progesterone in 200- and 400-mg suppositories, to be inserted once or twice daily for 12-14 days of the month. It may also be used in the vagina.

Tablets
Duphaston	*dydrogesterone 10mg*
Primolut N	*norethisterone 5mg*
Utovlan	*norethisterone 5mg*

Gel
Crinone	*progesterone 4%*

Injection
Depo-Provera	*medroxyprogesterone 150mg, injected into a muscle, lasts three months. It is excellent against the menopausal symptoms, but may not benefit either your bones or your arteries.*

There is a wonderful choice in competing brands of HRTand in the variety of ways in which you can take it. However, for some people HRT is unsuitable, because of health risks (see page 74) or unacceptable side-effects. These side-effects are considered in the next chapter.

Chapter 11

Hormone Replacement Therapy (HRT): Side-Effects

Approximately one woman in six develops tiresome, but usually transient, side-effects when she first takes HRT, while a very few may develop more serious symptoms. In most cases the risks are spotted in advance, and HRT is never started. The risks of cancer of the womb and of breast cancer have now been reassessed as more severe than was thought previously. While a brief period on HRT is unlikely to do any harm, more than a year should be avoided and the general anti-cancer ploys stepped up whether you are on HRT or not.

Case Study
Charlotte was 48 when the vasomotor symptoms of the menopause – the big 3: hot flushes, night sweats and palpitations – began. She found it impossible to concentrate on her work and was delighted when her doctor said he had the answer and prescribed a popular brand of HRT. For an initial period of two or three weeks, Charlotte was buoyed up by hope, expecting that her symptoms would vanish. Instead they barely altered and she developed a new set of symptoms, every bit as troublesome.

Oddly enough, these symptoms reminded her of how she felt in the first three months when she was expecting her son Gary, now a young man of 23. She felt nauseated, and vomited on two occasions; her breasts were swollen and tender; her abdomen felt bloated. She also noticed some brownish patches on her face. The nausea occurred less often when she took the tablets with a meal, and, as she had done during pregnancy, she kept to hand a stock of semi-sweet biscuits to nibble when she felt tired or it seemed a long time to lunch.

Charlotte also bought a sports bra, providing all-round support without constriction, and her friend Sue, who was keen on alternative medicine, suggested Evening Primrose Oil and the B vitamins, especially B6, pyridoxine. Charlotte's breasts became more comfortable over the next few weeks and the bloating improved over the same period, perhaps in part because she cut down on her six mugs of coffee daily.

Charlotte's experience of symptoms as her body adjusted to the changes in her hormone status was the norm. The extra oestrogen was responsible for the nausea and breast discomfort, the progestogen for the bloating. She was lucky in having withdrawal bleeds, replacing her periods regularly each cycle, from the second month. Several of her friends reacted to their changing hormonal situation with up to six months of spotting and break-through bleeding before their cycles settled into a regular rhythm.

While Charlotte's symptoms were little trouble and did not last, some-times they persist and it is then useful to know which component of the HRT, oestrogen or progestogen, needs adjusting.

Common Symptoms due to Oestrogen

Nausea
If taking the medication with meals or at bedtime does not resolve this, using a lower dose of oestrogen to start with may solve the problem. This involves taking separate oestrogen and progestogen tablets instead of one combination tablet, or else changing to a patch, which gives a lower dose.

Sore, Swollen Breasts
If a new bra does not help, it is worth cutting out all caffeine – coffee, tea, chocolate and cola drinks. The discomfort is only temporary.

Spotting and Breakthrough Bleeding
This is bleeding that appears at the wrong time in the cycle. It is very com-mon and nothing to worry about in the first six months after starting HRT, but is nonetheless annoying. It is not predictable, which means you must take precautions. Out-of-phase bleeding is especially liable to trouble those who have their change young, say in their early 40s, or who have begun HRT a year or less after their last period.

The answer is not in the no-bleed types of HRT. Even with these, unscheduled bleeding often occurs in the first months. Similarly this hap-pens with Tridestra, which runs in a three-month cycle instead of the usual one-month cycle.

Situations that Require Investigation
- Heavy bleeding: quite often this is caused by a fibroid in the uterus being stimulated by the oestrogen of HRT to grow larger and inciden-tally increase the area of womb lining that bleeds
- Irregular bleeding persisting for more than three or four cycles, or start-ing up after a an elapse of time with no bleeding.
- Discomfort or pain in the pelvis – this may be due to an infection in any of the organs in the area, for instance the bladder or the Fallopian tubes, or a fibroid may be undergoing degeneration. There is also the possibility that the pain is being caused by a tumour.

If investigations reveal nothing abnormal, the next step is similar to that for persistent nausea – trying a smaller dose of the oestrogen temporarily, or using a patch. Tablets provide a large input at one moment, then a gap with nothing until the next dose. This irregularity may, in itself, trigger the symptoms. With excessive or prolonged bleeding a test for anaemia is a must, to prevent your sinking into a low-energy, low-mood state.

Putting on Weight
Next to irregular bleeds, this is the commonest reason for giving up HRT after only two or three months. While it is true that many women put on weight at the time of their menopause, the cause is not HRT, but the physiological changes of this important phase in your life. Your metabolism slows down, so you need less food although your lifestyle may remain the same – but there is a tendency at 50ish to take less exercise. The mild increase in testosterone (male hormone) may encourage weight gain, particularly at the waist. Incidentally, it is testosterone that causes an increase in facial hair. This is usually negligible and can be dealt with by plucking out the odd offending whisker. Rarely, it calls for cosmetic treatment with depilatories or electrolysis.

HRT is not responsible for weight gain – as has been demonstrated by several large research studies. Women who take HRT were shown to put on less weight than women not taking HRT.

One fairly common cause of weight gain at this age, which is often overlooked, is an underactive thyroid (hypothyroidism). This is easily treated – once the situation is recognized.

However the unwanted flab arises, it is important for your heart and your self-esteem to lose the excess and then maintain the reduction. Exercise is one strand in the treatment of overweight (see page 47), but the unavoidable other one is calorie control.

The formula for assessing whether you are overweight is the BMI – Body Mass Index. It comprises your weight in kilograms divided by your height, in metres, squared. For example, a woman who weighs 57 kg (126 lb or 9 st) and is 1.6 metres tall (5 ft 4 inches) would figure out her BMI by dividing 57 by 2.56 (that is, 1.6 x 1.6), to come up with the number 22.

A healthy BMI is 20-25 for a woman, while a BMI of over 27 is considered obesity. If your BMI works out at 25-27, be careful – you are running towards danger, and 27-plus calls for action.

The big killer of post-menopausal women is coronary artery disease, related to overweight. While breast cancer is less likely before the menopause if you are plump, the risk after the change is greater. The risk of diabetes, high blood pressure and chest and joint problems increase with every extra pound. The bonus is slightly less susceptibility to osteoporosis.

Skin Disorders

Itching, skin irritation and rashes are among the common, non-serious and usually transient symptoms of the menopause, and in a few women patches of brown pigmentation appear, especially on the face. The first three are much more likely if you are taking your HRT in patches. Gels do not have this effect, but most people find it simpler to take tablets.

Hormone implants of oestrogen, progesterone or testosterone are usually trouble-free, but may work their way to the surface of the skin, especially the progesterone cylinder type. These cylinders leave tiny scars and, if you decide to stop using them, are difficult to remove.

While it is the oestrogen that underlies most of the common side-effects of HRT, progestogens are not entirely blameless.

Common Symptoms due to Progestogen

Side-effects often blamed on progestogen include:
● Bloating and other symptoms of the premenstrual syndrome
● Tender breasts
● Mood swings
● Depression
● Weight gain
● Headaches
● Acne

Bloating

This uncomfortable tightness in the abdomen is caused by a relaxation of the muscles of the gut wall, allowing the bowel to swell out. It is often part of the premenstrual syndrome and its cousin, irritable colon, as well as a side-effect of some types of progestogen. These include norethisterone, norgestrel and levonorgestrel. A change to medroxyprogesterone or dydrogesterone may help, and some sufferers find, through trial and error, that cutting out a particular food improves the situation. This is an individual matter, and there are no hard and fast guidelines.

Natural progesterone causes fewer side-effects. It may be given in a gel, directly into the vagina.
● Crinone: one applicatorful is inserted into the vagina on alternate days for the last 12 days of each cycle.

A novel method of giving a progestogen is in an IUD, an intrauterine device similar to the IUCD, the contraceptive. Since it acts directly on the womb lining, only a minute dose is required, hopefully one too small to cause side-effects.

- Mirena: a T-shaped device which is inserted into the womb and gradually delivers a small amount of levonorgestrel. It does not require replacing for five years. Several other gels and devices are being developed, but there are difficulties in getting these to provide an effective dose.

Since progestogens are often used for contraception, it is simple to add an oestrogen, in continuous dosage, to convert it to HRT at the appropriate time.

'Natural' Progesterone Creams

These creams have recently become very popular. They have been available over the counter in mainland Europe and the US for 20 years, and they are now available on prescription in the UK, although they are not yet generally licensed.

Natural progesterone is so-called because it can be made from several plants, including soya beans and yams; unlike the synthetic progestogens it is identical in chemical structure to our own woman-made progesterone. It has recently been promoted in the UK as a preventative and treatment for osteoporosis because laboratory studies have shown that progesterone stimulates the bone repair cells, the osteoblasts. Disappointingly, the result of applying the natural progesterone creams Pro-Gest and Pro-Juven is minuscule. The amount of progesterone delivered is not enough to have a measurable effect on bone loss, nor to counteract the influence of oestrogen-only HRT.

The good news is that these creams definitely help with the vasomotor symptoms of the menopause, as demonstrated in a trial lasting a year. The one side-effect, which applied to only a few women, was vaginal spotting, and this lasted only one to two days. However, these creams *must not be used* if you have a liver problem.

Breast Lumps

Breast lumps are frightening and often occur in the menopausal years. Nearly all of them are harmless, and come in two types: fibroadenomas and cysts. Cysts feel smooth and firm to the touch, while fibroadenomas are solid and hard. They consist of glandular and stringy fibrous tissue knotted together.

Both types are common and in themselves benign, but they are important because some of the cysts in particular may be the long-term forerunners of breast cancer. Cyst formation is stimulated by methylxanthine, a chemical found in coffee, tea, cola drinks, chocolate and also tobacco. Smokers are extra liable to cysts. One in 10 breast lumps may turn out to be cancerous – the older you are the more likely – so it is important to find them so that they can be dealt with.

One way of discovering a breast lump is by feeling your breast all over systematically; your doctor may do this. Mammograms and ultrasound examination reveal particularly small lumps. A needle biopsy (involving taking a tissue sample) can then be tested to check if the lumps are benign. The procedure known as breast aspiration is similar to biopsy, while a new electrical method for assessing the density of a lump is being developed to distinguish between harmless and malignant lumps.

Fibrocystic Disease
Also known as 'benign breast change', this affects more than one-quarter of women, but mainly before the menopause. It comprises fibrous thickening of the breast tissue with the development of multiple small cysts. It improves as the oestrogen level falls after the change.

Breast lumps matter because of the worry they cause, and the slightly increased cancer risk. Conventional treatments have little to offer, but vitamin B6 (pyridoxine) and Evening Primrose Oil may have some effect, as with Charlotte's rather different breast symptoms (see page 69).

Serious Side-effects

Those mainly associated with oestrogen:
● Cancer of the breast
● Cancer of the womb

Those associated with both oestrogen and progestogen:
● Deep vein thrombosis (DVT)
● Pulmonary embolism
● Eye problems

Those mainly due to progestogen:
● Acute liver problems
● Premenstrual tension
● Depression
● Insomnia, headaches, mood swings

Now we'll look at five of these in more detail: breast and womb cancer, DVT, acute liver problems, and depression.

Cancer of the Breast
This is the most common of women's cancers, and occurs more often in Great Britain than anywhere else in the world, but alarmist reporting

makes the danger sound worse than it is.

Who Is at Risk?
- Those already suffering from cancer of the womb or colon
- Those who have other family members with breast cancer, especially a mother, sister or aunt, especially if these relatives developed the disease before the age of 50, or if more than one relative has been affected
- High birth weight – another factor you cannot control
- Having had periods for 35 years or more
- Those who did not have children before the age of 30, or who've had no children at all
- Those with benign breast changes – but it may be 15 to 20 years before a cancer develops
- Those aged between 35 and 54, but especially past 50. Up to the menopause the breast cancer rate increases with age, but then it almost levels out
- Those exposed to radiation from any cause, for instance treatment for some other disorder
- Those who are overweight – this only applies when it occurs after the change
- Women who took the contraceptive pill for four years or more in their early 20s; there is no added risk for those who started taking the Pill in their late 20s onwards
- Women who have undergone severe emotional stress in the previous five years, including bereavement.

The Relation of Breast Cancer to HRT
The statistics are frustratingly inconclusive. What is known is that oestrogen taken by mouth protects against breast cancer. This is not the case with oestrogen patches. Also, the beneficial effect is cancelled by some progestogens, including levonorgestrel and norethisterone, both of which are derived from testosterone. Medroxy-progesterone and dydrogesterone do not have this effect.

Taking HRT for up to 10 years has an influence on the chances of breast cancer, after that the risk may increase by as much as 30% of the small average risk.

HOW MANY WOMEN ARE AFFECTED?
- Those not taking HRT   45 /1,000
- Taking HRT for 5 years   47/1,000
- Taking HRT for 10 years   51/1,000

● Taking HRT for 15 years   57/1,000
(but even after 15 years the risks are less than for women whose menopause came late naturally).

This slow increase in risk over time diminishes as soon as you stop the
HRT, and is cancelled completely after two to five years.

Prevention of Breast Cancer
SERMS (SELECTIVE (O)ESTROGEN RECEPTOR MODULATORS)
● Tamoxifen, an anti-oestrogen
● Raloxifene, used for osteoporosis
These are only used for those at special risk, because of their side-effects.
For example, tamoxifen may cause hot flushes, clotting and – rarely – pul-
monary embolism, a 1-in-1,000 increase in the risk of cancer of the womb,
cataracts and depression.

General Anti-cancer Measures
Eating plenty of fruit and vegetables, especially those
containing antioxidants including vitamins C, E and A
Taking regular physical exercise.

A note of cheer – if you are unlucky enough to develop cancer while you
are taking HRT, it is likely to be mild.

Cancer of the Womb
This is more accurately termed endometrial cancer (the endometrium is
the lining of the womb), to distinguish it from cancer of the cervix. Cervical
cancer usually affects younger women, and is not associated with the
menopause – unlike endometrial cancer. As the ovaries stop producing
eggs on a regular basis, the trigger for making progesterone is lost. This
means that the oestrogen still produced by the ovaries continues to stimulate the womb lining – unchecked. Adding an oestrogen-only form of
HRT quadruples the risk of a cancer developing – increasing with every
dose of oestrogen you take without the balancing effect of a progestogen.

Risk Factors for Endometrial Cancer
● Oestrogen alone or in HRT – taking a progestogen
   reduces the risk enormously
● Obesity
● Diabetes
● High blood pressure

The symptom that should alert you is bleeding from the vagina. If this occurs without a clear cause, it must be investigated, preferably including an ultrasound examination. The essential treatment is hysterectomy, followed, in some cases, by a radiation implant in the vagina to deal with any remaining cancer cells. The bonus after a hysterectomy is that there is no more worry about the effects of oestrogen without progestogen.

Case Study
Isobel had just started combination HRT when she was 53. She was worried when, a few months later, she began to be aware of a full feeling in her abdomen, which seemed definitely swollen. Then she had an alarmingly heavy bleed followed by irregular bleeding. Isobel was sure that she had cancer of the womb, and her doctor took her situation quite seriously. He carried out a clinical examination and found that Isobel's womb felt 'bulky'. Ultrasound revealed the cause as a cluster of fibroids.

These fibroids had obviously been there for some years, but had caused no trouble, and were shrinking as Isobel went into the menopause and her oestrogen levels declined. The dose of oestrogen in the HRT more than made up the deficit and stimulated the fibroids to grow and bleed excessively. Isobel stopped the HRT and had a hysterectomy to avoid any more trouble with her uterus. She was in hospital for four days, but it took six weeks for her to recover sufficiently to go back to her demanding job in fashion.

Isobel could then take oestrogen-only HRT and chose Premarin, a long-established preparation. She has been advised to remain on it for several years as insurance against osteoporosis.

Cancers of the Cervix and Ovary
These are common, but have no link with the menopause or HRT.

Deep Vein Thrombosis (DVT)
DVT is the formation of blood clots in the deeply-placed veins of the lower leg. While there is an increased risk, statistically, of DVT when you take HRT, this is still very small:
● 1 in 10,000 women develop DVT if they are NOT on HRT
● 3 in 10,000 develop it in the first year of taking HRT
● 6 in 10,000 develop it while pregnant.

It is to guard against DVT that you are given elastic stockings after your hysterectomy. The symptoms may be extremely slight, but include pain and swelling in the calf, and legs that feel warm to the touch.

Predisposing causes:

- Being immobilized, for example when in hospital or, as has made headlines of late, during the course of a long plane journey
- Increasing age
- Overweight
- Varicose veins
- Family history of the syndrome.

DVT is significant because it carries the risk of pulmonary embolism if a fragment of the clot gets carried away in the bloodstream and lodges in an artery in the lung. This can cause sudden death.

Acute Liver Problems

Jaundice, a yellowing of your skin and the whites of your eyes, is the unmistakable signal of a liver in trouble, and if you experience these symptoms you must stop taking HRT. Both the oestrogen and the progestogen in HRT increase the likelihood of gallstones, and if one of these blocks the bile duct it causes abdominal pain and jaundice. Processing the steroid element in HRT can throw a strain on the liver, so you should not take it if you have had any liver problems in the recent past.

Depression

Everyone who has suffered from a depressive illness contends that it is much worse than having a physical disorder. HRT has a reputation for lifting mood: this is due to the oestrogen. Progestogens can have the opposite effect, and this may be noticeable when they are introduced into your cycle. Higher doses of progestogen increase the depth of the depression: this is demonstrated by a low, miserable mood, lack of self-care, insomnia and poor concentration, and unreliable memory. The mornings are the worst time.

When depression means more than unhappiness or dissatisfaction with life, when you cannot eat and have lost weight, when sleep deserts you after 4 a.m. and you feel worthless, you probably need an antidepressant. One of the modern selective serotonin re-uptake inhibitors (SSRIs) related to Prozac is more suitable than the older, tricyclic types, as the latter can exaggerate mood swings in the menopause. Supportive psychotherapy – discussions to boost self-esteem – are a valuable adjunct to the medication.

Chapter 12

Exercise as Treatment

We are told that exercise is good for us – and this alone is a turn-off. In fact, between 30 and 50% of us would score nil for the amount of leisure-time physical exercise we took in the last month. Yet if you heard of anything else that would delay the ageing process, pep up your brain power and improve your looks – wouldn't you be queuing for it?

What Exercise Can Do forYou

- Avoid or improve osteoporosis
- Improve your heart and circulation, reducing the risk of heart attack and high blood pressure
- Reduce the risk of developing cancer – and give any treatment a boost
- Reduce the risk of developing diabetes
- Increase your muscle strength
- Loosen up your joints
- Increase the blood supply to your brain
- Help you to sleep soundly
- Put your worries in perspective
- Increase the circulation to your skin, acting like a tonic
- Boost your self-esteem
- Induce an all-over feeling of well-being

With all these benefits, how is it that so many of us short-change our bodies by taking so little exercise? In the UK and the US and other countries with a Western lifestyle, technology has robbed us of opportunities to exercise – at home we don't even have to get up to switch television channels, and at work we are often glued to a screen for hours, moving no more than a finger. We women are particularly lax in the matter of exercise. Among those of us between 50 and 64, the menopausal and postmenopausal years, fewer than half take any regular exercise, while women of 65-plus have a lower level of physical activity than any other group.

National guidelines on exercise are put out by both the US and UK Departments of Health, but the vast majority of people take no more notice of them than they do of the speed limits on our roads.

The Recommendations

Until recently we were advised to take a minimum of 30-60 minutes of moderate to vigorous exercise three times a week. This can be boring or difficult to fit in, so a modification has been introduced that is easier to comply with and more palatable. You achieve the same amount of exercise but in 10- to 15-minute chunks. Three 10-minute slots of brisk walking or aerobics daily is the minimum with this formula. It uses twice as much energy if you walk uphill or climb stairs, equivalent to any obviously vigorous exercise.

Whatever your programme, you need to incorporate it into your daily routine and keep it up. Nearly 70% of menopausal women drop out of an exercise routine that involves nothing more taxing than a walk. Don't be one of them.

The Effects

Age is no bar – and no excuse. Your body's response to exercise will be as good at 50, 60 or 70 as it would be if you were a trained athlete. The only difference is that you start from your own baseline level to achieve the same degree of benefit:

● Improved heart and lung function – 10 to 30%,
  measured by the amount of oxygen you use
● Increase of muscle strength by two or three times
● Increased range of movement in the large joints
● Increased flexibility.

These last three counteract the natural tendency, as you reach the menopausal and postmenopausal years, for your muscles to become weaker and your joints stiffer. Mobility is one of your most precious assets, and worth preserving.

Snags and Advantages

Smoking, overweight, heavy drinking, low income and higher age are linked to less exercise, while the golden girls – and boys – tend to exercise as a matter of course. The well-off, well-educated and younger women value and look after their bodies the best.

Not everybody benefits from exercise.

It is not for you if:
- You have recently had a heart attack
- Your electrocardiogram (ECG) shows some abnormalities or changes
- Your blood pressure is seriously high
- Certain heart disorders: heart block, valvular disease, irregular rhythm
- Diabetes or thyroid disease that is not well controlled
- Acute arthritis
- Severe osteoporosis

Help with Special Problems

Overweight
Of adults in their third to sixth decades, 33% are overweight. It is often the chief complaint of women in their perimenopause and later. A Body Mass Index (BMI) of 27 or more means a serious risk to health, with four times the risk of coronary artery disease, the top killer for women of this age (see pp 44-45). Fortunately, the perimenopause is a most propitious time for taking control of your weight. Diet and exercise are the only safe and effective methods of treatment.

Diabetes
The non-insulin-dependent Type 2 diabetes is forecast to increase by 16% in the next few years, largely because of the epidemic of overweight. The best preventative is exercise – even a moderate amount provides worthwhile benefits. Exercise also offers the following benefits:
- Allows for a decrease in insulin requirement
- Better control of glucose (sugar) level in the blood
- Lowering of blood pressure
- Lowering of cholesterol level, in particular the harmful LDL kind.

Exercise is particularly effective in the high risk group of overweight women with high blood pressure and a family history of diabetes. There is a 6% reduction in the risk of developing diabetes for every 500 calories burnt off by exercise.

Osteoporosis
Inactivity is one of the main causes of bone loss, and the best treatments are calcium, hormones and exercise.

Falls and Fractures
These are an increasing risk for women from age 60 onwards, and the common hip fracture carries a substantial danger of long-term crippling

and, indirectly, death. Exercise greatly reduces the risk of falls, even in the very frail and elderly. It acts by:

- Strengthening the bones
- Training and strengthening the muscles
- Improving reaction times
- Improving balance

Isometric muscle-strengthening exercises and walking are the most beneficial for this purpose. Isometric or anaerobic exercise involves tightening the muscles and holding the tension without moving the part. *Iso-* means 'the same', *-metric* means 'measurement'.

Cancer

The risk of colon cancer is greatly reduced by exercise. In The Nurses' Health Study of 1997, an hour a day of moderate exercise led to a decrease of 46% in the risk of developing cancer of the colon. This is probably due to the fact that exercise speeds up the transit time of the contents of the colon.

The situation regarding breast cancer is less clear: some trials show exercise as beneficial, some are inconclusive, but none is negative. The exercise some women take doing housework and looking after children may account for some of the differences.

Depression

This is a frequent cause of suffering among women around the time of the menopause. Exercise can help by improving the body image and raising self-esteem, reducing the severity of vasomotor symptoms, inducing physical relaxation and calming mild anxiety.

Adverse Effects of Exercise

These are few, and seldom serious. Overuse of the ankles and knees by runners and of the shoulder joints by swimmers can cause strains and sprains, while jarring of the bones and joints can result from jogging, running or jumping exercises. This can be harmful if you already have the beginnings of osteoporosis, which is likely as the menopause approaches and oestrogen levels decline. Similarly, overextending your spine or bending it forwards more acutely than is comfortable can damage any weakened vertebrae. Thick-soled shoes and avoidance of extremes help you to get the maximum benefit from your exercise safely.

In those with mild, unrecognized heart problems, exercise that is too vigorous may bring on angina, or upset the rhythm of the heartbeat. If you are about to undertake a course of exercise or to attend a gym, it makes good sense to have a physical check-up first. This will include your heart and circulation as well as your ankles, knees and back.

The perimenopausal years are crucial to your health, not just for now but for the rest of your life. This is a time to review your lifestyle and drop unhealthy habits that have sneaked in – such as too many cups of coffee, glasses of wine or chunks of chocolate – and lolling about in front of the television. You also need to establish some good habits – and taking regular exercise comes under this heading. The trick is to make it enjoyable – something you look forward to. Joining an aerobics class is one way of doing this, ringing the changes in your exercises is another, or exercising along to music or a talking book.

Types of Exercise

Aerobic
This means any kind that raises your heart rate and makes you 'puffed'. It includes exercises that you can do on your own, such as swimming, cycling, fast walking, jogging, running and jumping/skipping. In a gym there are treadmills, stationary bicycles and other apparatus which tell you your heart rate and the energy you are using.

Aerobics with other people can be fun, for instance in classes with music and an instructor, or in games like netball, tennis or badminton. Dancing can be a delight, and there is a wide choice – square, ballroom, Scottish, line and country varieties – now available.

Anaerobic or Isometric
This strengthens your muscles by increasing the tension in them, group by group. The muscles involved are the large ones – in your back, abdomen, thighs and calves.

Callisthenics
Greek for 'strength and beauty', callisthenics involve movements made without effort, gracefully performed: sit-ups, toe-touching, circling your arms, sideways bends, knee-ups and leg lifting. They are useful in the warm-up and cool-down phases of an exercise session, together with stretch exercises. There is an instinct to stretch when you first wake up, and it is helpful to emulate a cat to enjoy it.

Yoga is similar to callisthenics, although bear in mind that until you are proficient, the more extreme body positions may be unsuitable for you.

Structured Walking

This is safe and effective for anyone. Establish a 30- to 45-minute time frame every day or every other day. This period is then divided into three phases:

- Warm-up, lasting 5 – 10 minutes
- Aerobic phase of fast walking: you aim to achieve 60-90% of your maximum output and hold it for three or four minutes to start with, building up to a 30-minute stint. You can judge your output by your pulse. Your maximum heart rate per minute is 200 minus your age – that is, 150 at age 50.
- Cool-down, for 5-10 minutes, bringing you back to your starting point at a slow pace.

Everyday Exercises

These include such activities as shopping, housework, going up and down stairs, sweeping up leaves and dog-walking. They can be seen as an extra bonus or – if timed and moderately vigorous – count towards your overall exercise routine.

A Complete Exercise Programme

Every week:
- 2-3 sessions of isometric muscle-strengthening exercises
- 3-4 aerobic sessions

This is an ideal to aim for, and you may sometimes fall short. What is essential is to keep up the minimum, either 40-minute stints three times a week or a daily dose of 30-45 minutes of divided exercise. This can be 10 minutes of household chores plus 10 minutes walking to work and 10 minutes walking back in the evening – or whatever fits your circumstances.

Chapter 13

Treatment Other than HRT

Hormone replacement treatment with oestrogen covers a range of menopausal symptoms, but it is certainly not the only treatment available.

Vasomotor Symptoms

As you know from reading this book, these include hot flushes (or 'flashes' as they are called in the US), night sweats and palpitations, and they result from an upset of the thermo-regulatory system in the part of the brain called the hypothalamus. While this is most likely to be due to a fall in oestrogen levels because of the menopause, these symptoms can also crop up in cases of overactive thyroid and diabetes, or as an allergic reaction. If there is any doubt, such possibilities need to be excluded, usually with blood tests.

Menopausal vasomotor symptoms frequently begin at age 47 or 48, but may appear much earlier. A common starting time is in the week before a period. Your skin becomes hot and red in blotches, affecting your chest and neck first, then rising to include your whole face and head. Your skin is hot to the touch, your pulse speeds up and you may get the bumping sensation of palpitations. Drenching sweats tend to come in the night, disturbing your sleep.

The symptoms are likely to continue for about three years, but can last as long as 15, especially if they began as early as 39. Twenty-five per cent of women have the hot flush syndrome on and off for more than five years, and 15% rate their symptoms as 'very severe'. For others, they may be so mild that no treatment is needed.

Commonsense Methods You Can Apply for Yourself
- Make a note of anything that appears to trigger the symptoms – and avoid it.
- Cut down on alcohol, tea, coffee and cola drinks – they stimulate the circulation.
- Give up smoking, if you have not done so yet – nicotine is also stimulating and can precipitate a flush.
- Hot soup and hot drinks, especially on an empty stomach, bring on the symptoms immediately – so miss them out.

- Go for cool, shady places in summer: avoid the direct, hot sun.
- Keep your rooms cool and well ventilated, particularly your bedroom.
- Use cotton sheets and nightwear.
- Have loose clothes in removable layers, made of natural fibres.
- Keep your weight down – you don't want an overcoat of fat.
- Keep a little electric fan and a toilet water spray in your handbag, plus a pack of moist wipes for your hands.
- Don't hurry; let troubles and irritations flow over you. Don't get steamed up – stretch and take half a dozen deep breaths instead.

Phyto-oestrogens

Make sure to eat plenty of these. While 80% of us in the West get some menopausal symptoms, they affect only 10% of Japanese and Chinese women. This is believed to be due to the large proportion of phyto-oestrogens in their diet. These are natural oestrogen-like substances found in most plants. Extra rich sources include soya, linseed and the whole pea and bean family. However, it must be said that phyto-oestrogens are not yet fully understood, and at times work as anti-oestrogens.

Foods Supplying Phyto-oestrogens

alfalfa	*liquorice*	*aniseed*
mung beans	*apples*	*mushrooms*
barley	*oatmeal, oat bran*	*broccoli*
parsley root	*caraway seeds*	*peas*
carrots	*plums*	*cherries*
pomegranates	*chick peas*	*poppy seeds*
citrus fruits	*potatoes*	*cranberries*
red beans	*dahl beans*	*red wine*
French beans	*rhubarb*	*garlic*
rice	*ginseng*	*rye, wheat*
hops	*sesame seeds*	*lentils*
soya beans	*linseed*	*tea*

Medication for Hot Flushes
- Dixarit (clonidine): Two to three 25-mcg tablets, morning and evening
- Inderal (propranolol): Two to three 40-mg tablets daily

Side-effects
Dry mouth, constipation, slow heart beat, cold hands and feet, digestive upset, disturbed sleep

Interactions
Tricyclic antidepressants, tranquillizers and blood pressure drugs

Exercise
Swimming is particularly suitable – can help with hot flushes. It reduces feelings of stress, and levels out mood swings.

Mind Over Matter
When you are getting hot, concentrate your thoughts on snow, ice and cold rain.

Irregular Periods

These are one of the most tiresome symptoms, interfering with your plans in an unpredictable way and sometimes involving painful cramps. They usually start about four years before the menopause itself, and often the first sign is that the gap between periods gets shorter. They may become heavy and prolonged, and later they may be spaced out so that you may think they have stopped.

Causes of Irregular Bleeding from the Vagina
● Excessive exercise
● Severe weight loss
● Eating disorders
● Emotional upset, stress
● Polyps
● Fibroids
● Endometriosis, a disorder of the lining of the womb

These possibilities need checking out before putting the symptom down to the menopause, and in particular if you have bleeding after sexual intercourse, between periods or after a gap of months without one.

Treatment
● Iron tablets, with vitamin C (which helps their absorption)
● B vitamins
● Phyto-oestrogens
● Have at hand supplies of extra-absorbent pads or tampons

Medication
● *Ponstan* (mefanamic acid): this acts by inhibiting the production of prostaglandins, the chemicals in the womb lining responsible for both

the cramps and heavy bleeding. The beneficial effect of Ponstan is weak, however, and it may cause a digestive upset or a rash, in which case it must be discontinued. It interacts with aspirin, anti-clotting drugs, blood pressure medicines, lithium and steroids. Dosage: 250-mg capsules, two or three times a day, starting on the first day of the period, for three to four days.

- *Cyklokapron* (tranexamic acid): this controls blood loss by helping the blood to clot more effectively in the lining of the womb. This, too, may cause a digestive upset, and in rare cases an interference with colour vision, when it must be stopped. Dosage: Two to three 500-mg tablets, three or four times daily for three to four days when there is heavy bleeding. This reduces the flow by up to 50%.
- *Ibuprofen*, which is related to Ponstan, is available from pharmacists over the counter. It relieves the pain of cramps, but does not reduce blood loss, and its side-effects include bleeding in the stomach and digestive upset. Dosage: 200- to 600-mg tablets, to make up 1,200-1,800 mg daily in divided doses, during the period.

Whichever drug is used, review progress every three months, continuing the treatment as necessary if there are no ill-effects.

Surgical Treatment
This is only needed with intractable heavy blood loss. The choice is between removal of much of the endometrium (the lining of the womb) – known as TCER or endometrial ablation – and partial or total hysterectomy.

Trans-Cervical Endometrial Resection (TCER)

There are several variations of this. In a frequently used type, the procedure is carried out under local anaesthetic and consists of cutting away part of the endometrium with a laser beam, via the cervix. Other methods, for which a general anaesthetic is required, include radio waves and electro-diathermy. For the latter, a current is passed through a loop of wire which is introduced into the uterus. It removes the endometrium in strips.

Endometrial ablation is not suitable if there are fibroids in the womb or pelvic inflammatory disease, and the surgeons need special training in the technique. On the plus side, complications are rare – less than 5%. This compares favourably with the results of hysterectomy, with which there is a complication rate of 48%. Another advantage with this treatment is that it can be carried out on a day-case basis, or with one night only in hospital, instead of several days. You will be able to go back to work in three to four weeks, unless you have a very physical job, compared with six to eight weeks after hysterectomy. Unlike the situation after a hysterectomy, you must still take a progestogen after the ablation if you are having oestrogen, because a little endometrium remains. For the same reason, although a pregnancy is extremely unlikely, it is not outside the bounds of possibility.

Twenty per cent of women have no bleeding at all two to three years after TCER, and up to 60% have reduced loss. That leaves 20-40% not much improved, and the occasional one with worse symptoms.

Case Studies
Olive had always had a tendency to heavy periods, but when she was about 44 they grew worse, and more frequent into the bargain. She became severely anaemic and constantly felt exhausted, while the iron tablets gave her stomach pains and made her constipated. Her friends and even her GP suggested that she could rid herself of the problem once and for all by having a hysterectomy. Although she was not planning to have any more children – her three were now teenagers – Olive could not bear the idea of having her womb removed. It was, to her, the essence of being feminine.

Her GP referred her to a specialist to discuss the situation, and that is how Olive heard about endometrial ablation. Unfortunately, this option was not available in her area. The nearest hospital which undertook this specialized surgery was some 50 miles away, and even if she had paid for private treatment locally it would not be in a hospital where the operation was routine and the staff well-versed in it. In the end, because it meant so much to her, Olive was accepted for treatment in a distant unit whereTCER by laser was practised.

Olive was nervous, so she was glad to have a general anaesthetic, sleep it off in hospital and leave the next day. The whole procedure went like clock-work, and although her abdomen was sore for several days, pain-killers kept this in check and she was pleased to be back home. After one heavy bleed, the aftermath of the operation, Olive's periods were considerably lighter, but she had to continue with iron supplements for several months. She tried the following slow-release iron preparations:
- Ferrograd: One 325-mg tablet daily
- Slow-Fe: One to two 160-mg tablets daily

Either of these minimized her stomach discomfort.

Olive was concerned that her motions were black, but her doctor explained that this was a normal effect of the iron.

Olive had a leaning towards alternative therapies, but decided, when her periods were petering out, to start on HRT for the sake of her bones and heart. Since she still had a uterus, she had to have a progestogen with the oestrogen. Olive is happy with her choice of TCER.

Pamela had got to know Olive at the surgery – she was a few years older, 49. She had a similar problem with excessive blood loss, but felt differently. Pamela was a down-to-earth person and thoroughly fed up with heavy, uncontrollable bleeding every month, and her lack of energy. She was only too glad to think that if she had a hysterectomy she would never have another period or even have a smear test. She discussed it with her husband, her doctor and her friends before making up her mind to have this major operation, and it was booked for two months' hence.

Pamela made good use of the waiting time by losing a few surplus pounds and working through a course of exercises, with special reference to the abdominal muscles. The hysterectomy went without a hitch, but Pamela had one of the common adverse effects – a urinary infection. At first she could not pass water, then she wanted to all the time and it burned. A short course of antibiotics dealt with the problem in a few days.

Pamela was able to leave hospital five days after the surgery, but was surprised how weak she felt. It was important not to put a strain on the healing wound, and she did not go back to her job (as a bookshop manager) for eight weeks. Olive felt superior, having taken only three weeks off work, but Pamela had no regrets about her choice.

Hysterectomy

100,000 hysterectomies are performed in the UK every year, and one woman in 5 of all those over 55 has been through the operation. Far the most common reason is excessively heavy periods, often with painful cramps: menorrhagia.

There are various types of operation: Vaginal or Abdominal, and Partial, Total or Radical.

Vaginal Hysterectomy
This is performed through a cut through the top of the vagina, from the inside. The uterus, including the cervix, is removed, leaving no external scar. It is the procedure of choice in prolapse of the womb, but is technically tricky, particularly if there are fibroids. Currently only about 12% of hysterectomies in the UK are done using this method, but it is becoming increasingly popular, especially in the US.

The advantages, apart from the absence of scarring, include less postoperative pain and a much quicker recovery time than with the standard abdominal operation. The hospital stay is reduced to two to four days, and complete recovery to within eight weeks.

Abdominal Hysterectomy

This is the standard approach, through an incision along the 'bikini line' at the lower border of the abdomen. It is the easiest for the surgeon and gives him or her the best view of the internal organs. However, there is more trauma to the tissues in total using this route, and the complication rate is high, at 42%.

Time Scale
In hospital: 4-6 days
Convalescence and recovery: 8 – 10 weeks,
sometimes as long as 12 weeks
Driving: 4-5 weeks, that is when the scar is pain-free
Sex: 5 weeks
Heavy lifting – shifting furniture, etc: 8 weeks

Types of Abdominal Hysterectomy

All involve an incision in the abdomen and a general anaesthetic.

Partial Hysterectomy
Removal of the body of the uterus, but preserving the cervix. There is an idea around that having a cervix increases your enjoyment of intercourse, but there is no evidence for this. Sexual feelings depend more on your relationship with your partner and your own self-confidence than on any type of hysterectomy – once the scars have healed and they are not tender. The disadvantage of leaving the cervix is that it remains a cancer risk, and you have to continue with smear tests. Partial hysterectomy is not recommended by gynaecologists.

Total Hysterectomy
This is what Pamela had, and it means removal of the whole of the uterus, but not the Fallopian tubes or ovaries. This gives you the best of both worlds – no periods, no smear tests and no risk of cancer of the womb, while the ovaries continue to produce hormones, only at a reduced rate as the menopause develops.

Menopausal problems come on immediately if both ovaries are removed, and these are particularly severe in younger women – in their early and mid-40s. If one ovary, or even a part of one is saved, the impact is much less. Normally, as in Pamela's case, the ovaries are left undisturbed by the hysterectomy. The reasons for removing them are unconnected with the menopause: they include ovarian cysts, a strong family history of cancer of the ovary, and endometriosis.

It is to the ovaries, not the womb, that we owe our femininity, but other

91

sources of oestrogen (be they natural or in hormone replacement therapy) make even the ovaries irrelevant. You may feel a sense of bereavement, that you have lost something precious after a hysterectomy, but this is a psychological reaction without a physical basis.

Very occasionally, severe, ongoing premenstrual tension (PMS) may make a woman decide to have her healthy ovaries removed.

Radical Hysterectomy
This involves resection of – cutting out – the uterus and cervix, the tubes, ovaries and lymph glands in the pelvis. The usual reason for this operation is a cancer in the area, when a 'clean sweep' is the safest option.

Complications which May Follow Hysterectomy
● Pain taking longer than usual to settle
● Deep vein thrombosis (DVT) – the risk is less with a vaginal than an abdominal operation, but more as you get older and if you are over-weight, have varicose veins, and undergo a prolonged stay in hospital for whatever reason
● Difficulty in passing water can follow any gynaecological operation, and may be due to local pain and swelling of the tissues, urinary infection or certain drugs (anticholinergics, including antidepressants)
● Urinary infection, causing pain on passing water, frequency, urgency and a fever
● Infection in the wound
● Haematoma – a leakage of blood collecting in the wound
● Chest infection, particularly in the elderly, smokers, overweight people or those with a painful scar who are afraid to breathe deeply

A slight rise in temperature is a normal reaction to surgery

Vaginal Dryness

This is a very common, almost universal, symptom of the menopause. With the reduction in oestrogen, the membrane lining the vagina becomes thinner and less elastic, in fact more delicate. There is also less of the fluid which lubricates it, and its chemical make-up alters. The vagina can become sore and itchy, even burning. One effect of this is discomfort during intercourse – *dyspareunia* – while another is having to pass water frequently, and urgency – you cannot wait. The urine tube, the urethra, is lined with the same epithelium as the vagina, and is equally liable to irritation.

Simple Manoeuvres to Combat Vaginal Dryness

- Avoid bubble baths, scented soaps and shower gels – keep to soaps and detergents suitable for babies.
- Wear loose cotton – or silk – underwear, no man-made fibres.
- If you wear jeans, make sure they are not tight in the crotch.
- Wear stockings or pop socks rather than tights.
- Have plenty of foreplay before intercourse to stimulate lubrication, and try to have sex regularly – remember 'if you don't use it, you lose it.'
- Use KY jelly to help lubrication.
- Apply live natural yoghurt to increase the acidity of the natural lubrication – this helps to prevent thrush.
- Vitamin E and Evening Primrose Oil may help.

Oestrogen creams, pessaries, rings and tablets are also used to treat vaginal dryness: see pp 17, 19, 20.

Vaginal Infection: Vaginitis

The changes in the lubrication of the vagina make it more susceptible to infection.

- Thrush – also called candida or moniliasis – is caused by a very common fungus. It causes itching and burning, sometimes amounting to pain and even bleeding, and a white discharge. Treatment: nystatin cream or pessaries; clotrimazole (Canesten) cream or pessaries; or fluconazole (Diflucan) capsules, 1 daily.
- Trichomonas vaginalis (TV) – produces irritation in and around the vagina, as with thrush, and a copious yellowy-green discharge which smells unpleasant. Metronidazole (Flagyl) pessaries and tablets deal effectively with this, but it is important not to drink any alcohol, as it interacts with the drug.

Urinary System Infections

Local oestrogen preparations often improve symptoms affecting the urethra, but if there is a urinary infection with burning on passing water, frequency and a raised temperature, an antibiotic is needed:

- Nitrofurantoin (Furadantin): One 50-mg tablet four times a day for seven days, or
- Nalidixic acic (Negram): One or two 500-mg tablets four times a day for seven days, then reducing to three times daily until the condition has cleared up.

It also helps to drink plenty of water.

Chapter 14

AlternativeTherapies

Traditional medicine can work wonders – for instance with antibiotics for pneumonia, or hip-replacement for arthritis. The menopause comes into a different category from straightforward physical disease. Although there may be physical symptoms, it is not an illness but a stage in life which involves hormonal, emotional and physical changes. Every corner of the body and mind is affected.

Hormone replacement therapy is the best treatment we have, but it compensates to some extent for the fall-off in only one hormone, oestrogen. The experience of hot flushes, sweats and palpitations, and often feeling generally out of sorts, can start long before your periods peter out and may linger on for years afterwards. A tendency to depression or anxiety can pervade your thinking and feeling, and your mood may vary unpredictably. Fatigue may be linked to anaemia, but is just as likely to sweep over you for no reason, and your sleep may be patchy and unrefreshing.

A lot of what you suffer is vague and difficult to pinpoint – and not merely a matter of chemistry. Altogether you need something to help you through the bad days, either to relax or to invigorate you and make you feel better in yourself.

This is where alternative or complementary therapies come in. These terms are two aspects of non-conventional medicine – alternative if you use it *instead* of orthodox treatments, *complementary* if you use it as an extra, or to fill in the gaps. Either way, the object is gently and safely to build up your general health and sense of well-being.

There is an enormous diversity of treatments – to suit every personality and alleviate a wide range of symptoms, especially those without a clear physical cause but no less distressing because of that.

Tranquillizers, sedatives and antidepressants manufactured by the pharmaceutical companies seldom help in the menopause, and may even make you feel worse because of their side-effects. By contrast, some alternative treatments may rescue you from the physical and emotional doldrums of this time of life. A herbal or homoeopathic medicine or a course of acupuncture may help. The one essential ingredient in all alternative therapies is time – time to listen to your body, to what you think and feel, what you believe is the cause of your symptoms and what sort of treatment you would like.

The alternative therapist is not working against the clock, with a waiting room full of patients, some of them with urgent problems. Because you, personally, are paying the fee you know your therapist is working for you, not for the hospital, the NHS or a Government target. You and he – or she – are working together as equal partners in the important task of helping you to get the best out of your life.

The great disadvantage of alternative therapy is that in a serious or life-threatening situation the gentle, indirect approach is ineffective. A lesser snag is that the cost may put it out of the reach of many ordinary people, particularly if a long course of treatment is needed. Twenty sessions would not be unusual; the Alexander technique, for example, requires 30 or 40.

Self-help

What you can do on your own is seldom enough by itself, yet it underpins all other treatment. Some of the practical measures that don't need a therapist's help are described on page 119, and others are lifestyle issues. They involve ensuring adequate amounts of food for the body and nourishment for your mind, enough exercise, sleep, relaxation and stimulus. You also need to construct a support system of friends and relatives with whom you keep in touch and from whom you can receive help and understanding on a reciprocal basis.

Counselling

This is the simplest therapy to involve another person. He or she will listen while you talk about your physical and other problems, and your fears, hopes and things you find stressful. A counsellor will give you support and encouragement as you explore ways of coping now, and avoiding similar pitfalls in the future. He or she should not be expected to act as a skilled psychotherapist. Most GPs have counsellors attached to their surgery and a few sessions can help you put your problems in perspective.

Naturopathy

It was in the 18th century that Jean-Jacques Rousseau led the 'back-to-Nature' movement which has flourished ever since. He was appalled at the spreading pollution of the newly industrializing cities of Europe and believed that the key to human health and happiness lay in a state of nature. This was distilled into exposure to the healing powers of fresh air and sunlight, and a simple diet which we now consider to be the ideal. It was near-vegetarian, with very little fat or sugar and, of course, none of the caffeine-containing stimulant drinks we take so freely today. Vincent Preissnitz, a near contemporary of Rousseau, prescribed walks in the wild for his patients, through meadows and woods and by rivers. This was the cure for all sickness, so it was believed.

Conventional medicine, especially pharmaceutical drugs, were and are condemned by the naturopaths. Vitamins, on the other hand, are approved and recommended. Naturopathic therapists, with such a wide-ranging remit, have an answer to every health problem, from headaches to cancer, usually involving an overhaul of the way you live. You must not hope for quick results, but for the slow development of a happy body in a contented mind. Menopausal and other symptoms slip into perspective.

Homoeopathy

This is another complete system of healing which is still popular today. The ancient Greeks practised a simple version, but it was a German doctor, Samuel Hahnemann (1755-1843), who formulated its rules and laws and put it on the map.

The Rules
1. If a symptom is suppressed but not eradicated it will reappear, sometimes in a different area.
2. During recovery, symptoms will improve in the reverse order to that in which they arose originally.
3. An illness must always get worse before it gets better.

The Laws
1. The Law of Similars: 'like cures like' – for instance, a purge, in small doses, will cure diarrhoea, or a yellow plant will benefit a case of jaundice.
2. The Law of Infinitesimals: the more a remedy is diluted, the more powerful its effect, even to the point where not a single molecule of the original remedy remains in any given dose.

Another important principle in homoeopathy is matching the treatment to the life experience of the sufferer. Recounting your life history for this purpose is probably therapeutic in itself. Another plus for homoeopathic treatment is that the medicines cannot possibly have side-effects.

Massage

This is the archetypal hands-on treatment. At its simplest it involves stroking, rubbing and kneading, mainly of the muscles. The results are not confined to the parts which are treated, but have a whole-body effect, and the relaxed muscles induce a relaxed state of mind. The basic massage techniques were developed in Sweden and later in the Esalen Institute in California. The touch is light and soothing.

Deep tissue work means more vigorous handling. It may hurt at the time, but you feel great afterwards, with a renewed sense of vitality.

Chiropractic
The essence of this is manipulation of the spine, it always includes a sharp cracking sound. The theory is misalignment of the vertebrae causes not only muscle and joint pain but a variety of problems all over the body such as may plague you in the menopause. Correction of the displacement of the bones automatically alleviates the other problems. Chiropractic produces quick and often successful results, but they may not last.

Osteopathy
This well-established, respected treatment also involves manipulation but it is not limited to the backbone and there is no obligatory 'crack'. It is linked with naturopathy, and some practitioners are expert in both. Its effects are less immediate than with chiropractic, but they last longer. The manipulations are slower and more deliberate. While osteopathy is frequently used for muscular and joint pain, other bodily tensions and aches also benefit.

Aromatherapy
This method is currently the most popular form of massage. It involves the external use of various essential oils, derived from plants such as cypress, lavender, rose, geranium and clary (clear-eye). The oil must be diluted 6:10 with a bland base oil, for example almond or sunflower seed, before it can be applied to the skin. The oils can be massaged into the skin, sprinkled in a bath or footbath, made into a compress or inhaled from a burner. Rose oil, however it is used, is said to be good for vaginal dryness; cold compresses with lavender help with hot flushes; clary has a reputation for benefiting night sweats.

Aromatherapy is used in a range of disorders, from depression to muscle spasms, with different combinations of oil chosen to suit each situation. The aromas are believed to release endorphins in the brain, nature's home-produced pain-killers.

Reflexology
The theory behind this pleasurably soothing foot massage is that different zones of the body are mapped out on the soles of the feet, and manipulating these provides a method of treating distant organs. Irregular periods and

irritable colon are among the many disorders reflexology claims to help.

St John's Massage
This variation concentrates on the tendons rather than the muscles, and is particularly good for a stiff neck, whether psychologically caused or brought on by strain or exposure to draught. Tension headaches also benefit from this type of massage.

SOMA
This type of massage specifically aims to provoke 'body memories' and a release of emotion. It should be accompanied by a course of psychotherapy – talking treatment.

Shiatsu or Acupressure
This employs a Chinese massage technique, using the same meridians (lines of power) as acupuncture. The therapist stretches and presses the tissues using his or her fingers, thumbs, palms, elbows, knees and feet. In Japan, Shiatsu therapists are usually drawn from the blind, and this work is reserved for them. It requires extra sensitivity in the fingertips.

Rolfing
Rolfing lies somewhere between massage and osteopathy. Its aim is to help the body resist the force of gravity, which tends to pull it into a stoop or slouch after any event that disturbs the perfect upright posture. Ida Rolf believed that the outer 'skin' of the muscles, the *fascia*, gets pulled out of shape by the force of gravity, with far-reaching mental and bodily effects. The manipulations of Rolfing are designed to correct this. Later forms of this treatment include movements learned by the patient.

Movement Therapies

All massage techniques are geared to banishing pain and malfunction anywhere in the body, and to soothe or invigorate according to need. The other main branch of bodywork is movement – likely to appeal to the more dynamic personalities as opposed to those who prefer the more passive forms of massage.

T'ai Chi
This popular activity comprises a rhythmic cycle of exercises like a slow, gentle dance without stretching, strain, tension or any specific postures. It is best learned and practised in a class. Patience and perseverance are two of the lessons t'ai chi can teach us.

Yoga

This 3,000-year-old Indian therapy brings body and mind into harmony with each other and incorporates movement and posture. It can be performed so gently that even the very frail can benefit, but there are also more advanced exercises. It is especially useful in treating anxiety and high blood pressure, but many people with no specific problems attend regular classes to keep fit.

Case Study

Felicity was 60. She was depressed, sleeping badly, with no appetite and feeling that everything worthwhile in her life was over. Her job at the local hospital was made redundant when the hospital closed down. The chances of another job were zero. HRT might have helped, but her unstable high blood pressure ruled that out, with the added risk of total deafness if her otosclerosis got worse.

Felicity's doctor gave her the favourite antidepressants – Prozac (fluoxetine) and Tryptizol (amitriptyline) – but one made her feel anxious and the other clashed with her blood pressure medicine. Even if she took an aspirin, you could guarantee that Felicity would have side-effects. She needed an alternative to drugs.

It was not a cure, but Felicity felt a great deal better after she joined a yoga class. She could manage the exercises without strain, either to her limbs or her blood pressure. The added bonus was that she made new friends with her classmates, and the cost for a weekly class was no strain on her purse.

Rolfing Movement Integration and Hellerwork

Joseph Heller was a follower of Ida Rolf and added training in correct movements to the treatment – this was Hellerwork. Later the Rolf Institute developed its own movement programme. Either of these therapies is beneficial to chronically painful states, but there are no quick results.

Tragerwork

Named after Dr Milton Trager, this method relies on rhythmic rocking of the neck, trunk and limbs and brings on a feeling of lightness and fluidity. It is not helpful where there are more distressing symptoms.

The Alexander Technique

An Australian actor, Frederick Alexander kept losing his voice and then found that he was holding his body tensely and in a way that impeded his breathing. The technique he worked out to overcome this is now a well-respected method of treatment. Instruction and gentle hands-on guidance enable you to give up ugly habits of bad posture and develop easy, graceful ways of managing your body, including breath control.

The Alexander technique is useful in all stress-related problems such as menopausal palpitations and insomnia.

Feldenkrais
Moshe Feldenkrais was a physicist who had a theory about the integrated action of the nerves, muscles and bones that controls movement. In particular he stressed that movements occur in three dimensions, and developed exercises accordingly. These can be learned in a class. Feldenkrais is particularly useful when chronic tension is causing symptoms.

Acupuncture

This treatment is thousands of years old. Acupuncture is used for all kinds of pain, including tension headaches and migraine, pain associated with fibroids or periods, and low backache.

A course of 10 sessions is standard for assessing whether the treatment is going to work – if so, it can continue to 20 or more. Some acupuncturists say that you need three months' treatment to see if acupuncture will help.

The Procedure
The therapist starts with a series of questions about your physical health, your emotional state, and your family, home and work background. He or she will examine your tongue and your pulse minutely and may also feel your abdomen. A plan is then made and the treatment begins. This consists of inserting very fine disposable needles either superficially or 1-3 inches deep, then twisting or heating them or passing an electric current to intensify the effect. The needles remain in place for 20-40 minutes.

Side-Effects
These may include small bruises where tiny blood vessels have been punctured; and occasionally a flare-up of your symptoms, which may last several days, but no more. You must not have acupuncture if you are taking an anti-clotting medicine such as warfarin or heparin, because of the risk of internal bleeding.

The medicines that are used with alternative and complementary treatments are – naturally – herbal (see Chapter 15).

Chapter 15

Herbal Medicines

Plants have been used for food and medicine since time immemorial. The ancient civilizations – Egyptian, Greek, Aztec, Ayurvedic and Chinese – all had *materia medica*, lists of established remedies, nearly all of which were derived from plants. Many of our most frequently used medicines today also come from plants: digitalis (foxglove) for the heart, morphine (poppies) for pain, quinine for malaria and dill for babies with wind.

Latterly the great pharmaceutical companies have dominated the medical scene, but in the last few decades there has been a resurgence of interest in herbal medicine. This has been led by ordinary people seeking treatments that are more user-friendly and less invasive than the powerful chemical drugs, with their often unpleasant side-effects.

Phyto-oestrogens

These are substances found in plants which have effects similar to those of oestrogen but in a much weaker form. It is striking that in China and Japan and some other Asian countries, where the normal soy-based diet is rich in phyto-oestrogens, menopausal symptoms such as hot flushes and vaginal dryness and even osteoporosis are seldom seen. Yet these problems pose a substantial risk for women in the West who eat fewer plant oestrogens.

Phyto-oestrogens come in 10 groups, of which the most relevant to us are the *flavonoids*. They occur in most fruits, vegetables and cereals. *Isoflavones* are a flavonoid group that come from legumes, the pea and bean family.

Genistein
Genistein is an isoflavone found only in soya. It blocks the effects of natural oestrogen, reducing the risk of breast cancer, and it may even reverse the development of a cancerous tumour by interfering with its blood supply. Genistein helps with hot flushes, sweats, poor sleep and vaginal dryness. Genistein, a plant or phyto-oestrogen is believed to block the stimulating effect of natural oestrogen on human breast cancer cells specifically and to interfere with the blood supply to the tumour. Genistein also helps alleviate such menopausal symptoms as hot flushes, sweats, vaginal dryness and poor sleep. Phyto-oestrogens are very different chemically from natural oestrogen. That usually refers to animal, especially

human, oestrogen but horse oestrogen is regularly used in HRT and the pill.

Daidzein
This is another isoflavone found in soya products. It is not as useful as genistein with the specific symptoms of the menopause, but it slows down the ageing process including of arthritis, heart disease and cataracts.

Lignans
Lignans have both oestrogenic and anti-oestrogenic effects, depending on the dose – the amount in your food. They are found mainly in linseed (flax seed) but are also in other whole grains and berries.
Phyto-oestrogens are part of our food rather than medicine, but many health-food shops now carry isoflavones in 750-mg capsules. Phyto-oestrogens are probably better absorbed in foods, however, and it is certainly more natural when they are eaten in tofu or some other food source.

When and How to Use Herbal Medicines in the Menopause

Hot Flushes
Agnus Castus
This dried ripe fruit or crushed root of the Chaste tree provides a mix of flavonoids, glycosides, bitters and oils. It is the most effective herbal treatment for hot flushes and is also helpful in the premenstrual syndrome.
   Dosage: Two 3-mg tablets, three times a day – but not if you are taking a progestogen, since Agnus castus boosts natural progesterone production.

Black Cohosh
This also relieves hot flushes, and peps up your energy, calms your mood and improves depression. It is an effective medicine, but there are two snags: it increases flooding (excessive bleeding in a period), and there is doubt about whether it increases the small risk of breast cancer if taken long term. A limit of six months is suggested.
   Dosage: 40-200 mg daily of the dried root, or 2-4 ml of the extract.

Black Haw (Sweet Viburnum)
This relaxes the womb and the gut, and controls flooding or loose motions. It is helpful in painful periods and breast discomfort.
   Dosage: Capsules of the powder or a decoction taken three times a day.
Hawthorn Flowers and Leaves
These can be mixed with hops in a ratio of 4:1 and made into a tea – an old Wessex remedy for hot flushes.

Damiana
Damiana can be taken as a tea or in a capsule for flushes; it is also an anti-depressant and aphrodisiac!

Lime flowers, Motherwort and Wild Carrot
These can be used, in equal meaures, to make a tea.
   Other herbal preparations that may relieve hot flushes are Goldenseal, Lobelia, Mistletoe, Rue, Sarsaparilla, Wild Yam, and Shepherd's Purse. Dong Quai and Evening Primrose are often recommended, but there is no evidence that they have any effect on hot flushes.

Night Sweats
These often go with hot flushes and – again – *Agnus castus* is the most successful of the treatments available. Cold teas are often helpful. *Lady's Mantle* and *Horsetail* are the main ingredients in several of these teas, and *Golden Sage* is also recommended.
   Cold compresses made with extracts of linseed, chickweed or chamomile, most herbal teas, and aromatic oils, well diluted, are all suitable. Vitamin E in doses of 200-400 international units daily may be helpful, but takes three or four weeks to become effective.

Vaginal Dryness
There are several helpful preparations to insert directly into the vagina:
● Live yoghourt or *lactobacilli* in tablet form stimulate the vaginal secretions and increase their acidity. This wards off thrush.
● Aloe vera, calendula and comfrey have a similar effect, and discourage any infection in the vagina or the urine. They also damp down itching. They should be applied three times a day for three months. Oil of Evening Primrose and lavender oil, diluted, can be smeared inside the vagina and are both soothing and antiseptic. A warm douche of Goldenseal is particularly comforting.
● Motherwort and Agnus castus taken by mouth – 15 drops of extract in a glass of water three times daily – or Rosemary tea may improve the uncomfortable lack of lubrication, and incidentally help with headaches or a low mood.

Insomnia
This is often caused by night sweats. There are several ways of tackling it.
   In the bath: Clary sage or Lavender oil
   Vaporization of aromatherapy oils
Medicines by mouth:
● Passion flowers in white wine

- Valerian
- Lime flowers
- Jamaican Dogwood
- Lemon Balm: the diarist, John Evelyn, writing in 1624, praised this as 'sovereign for the brain. It strengthens the memory and powerfully chases away melancholy.'
- Maria Treben tea: this contains Cowslip, Lavender, St John's Wort, Valerian and Hops. You sip a warm cupful just before going to bed. Hops tend to turn off your sexual feeling, and cause skin irritation.
- Dr Vogel's sleeping drops: equal parts of balm, oats, Passion flower, Hops and Valerian. The dose, at bedtime, is 10 – 15 drops. Alternatively, you may use a herb pillow.

Menopausal Headaches
- Tea made with Raspberry leaves, Skullcap and Agnus castus in equal parts – a heaped teaspoonful of the powdered mixture is used in a cupful of boiling water, steeped for 5-15 minutes and drunk freely.
- Feverfew: 1-4 fresh leaves, taken in mashed banana or a bread sandwich to moderate their acrid taste; or one 125-mg tablet daily.

Depression, Anxiety and Mood Swings
- Panax ginseng is the most popular treatment for the psychological ills of the menopause. It can be taken as tablets or capsules, each containing 150 mg, three times a day, or as tea made from a quarter of a teaspoonful of the powdered root per cup. Taking Vitamin E enhances the effect of ginseng, but large doses of Vitamin C reduce its effect.
- Vervain was considered sacred by the Greeks and Romans, and has been used ever since as a treatment for depression and – particularly – anxiety, either phobic or the paranoid type in which the sufferer feels everyone is her enemy.
  Dosage: 5-10 ml of the tincture in water, three times a day.
- St John's Wort (Hypericum) is accepted even by traditional physicians as a reasonably good treatment for depression, with few side-effects. It is mildly sedative and may affect drivers. There are various preparations, but the standard British Herbal Pharmacopoeia tincture is taken in doses of 2-4 ml, three times daily.
- Chamomile (Roman type) is tranquillizing, particularly if you feel irritable, and useful in combating indigestion. It is often given with Valerian, Passion flower or Liquorice. The tincture is used in 5-10 ml doses. It makes an excellent, pleasant-tasting tea.
- Alfalfa (Lucerne) has an especially rich content of minerals – calcium, magnesium, phosphorus and potassium – and vitamins – A, B6, C, D,

E and K. It is believed to improve both physical and psychological well-being. It is available in 250-mg capsules to take three times a day, with meals, or as the 'green drink' made by passing the leaves through a blender.

Bach Flower Remedies

Dr Edward Bach, a fashionable Harley Street doctor until 1930, found, like Dr Preissnitiz (see page 96) that there were healing properties to be found in the countryside. Bach took dew from the flowers and also soaked their petals in spring water to produce at first 12, but finally 38 flower remedies to suit every personality and every emotional state. He believed they triggered the body's own healing powers. The theory, shared with homoeopathy, is that substances leave a kind of imprint where they have once been. Bach's remedies are still popular, particularly for menopausal and post-menopausal psychological upsets.

The Rescue Remedy
This combines Star of Bethlehem, Impatiens, Cherry, Plum, Clematis and Rock Rose. It is used in emotional crises, when the mind is numb, in turmoil or in a state of panic.

Homoeopathic Remedies for Menopausal Symptoms

- Lachisis: South American snake venom
- Pulsatilla (Wild Anemone): a herb that relaxes the mind, especially in women, and is mildly sedative
- Sepia: cuttlefish ink.

Herbs Thought to Be Useful in Oestrogen Deficiency

Agnus Castus	Black Cohosh	Black Haw	Broom
Clivers	Goldenseal	Lady's Mantle	Life root
Lime flowers	Marjoram	Motherwort	Nettles
Oats	Parsley	Pennyroyal	Raspberry leaf
Sage	St John's Wort	Valerian	

Herbs Found to Be Useful in Flooding

Bayberry bark	Beth root	Black Haw	Blue cohosh
Broom	Cranesbill	Goldenseal	Greater Periwinkle
Lady's Mantle	Raspberry leaf	Shepherd's Purse	Yarrow

Chapter 16

Sex and the Menopause

There is a scare story around that says that when a woman has her first hot flush or hits 50, her love life is over – that she cannot cope with sex and is no longer attractive to men. This is total rubbish. We all know that from 20 to 40 sexual activity and making babies holds a prominent place in many women's lives and thoughts. But the capacity to give and receive affection between the sexes, both physically and emotionally, is undiminished through to 80-plus, although the style may be modified. In their 50s, women claim to think about sex more often than they did 10 years earlier. This may be in part because they worry more about it, but they really shouldn't have to.

The fall-off in sexual intercourse that undoubtedly affects many women in this age group is often due, not to any physical or psychological deficiency in the woman, but to the lack of a partner. Men have a dangerous propensity to develop coronary disease from their 40s, unlike women either before the menopause or when they are taking HRT. Some women find themselves widowed young, or lose out in the game of change-partners, either at the first or second divorce. Others have husbands whose sexual prowess has taken a nose-dive. Sildenafil (Viagra) can rescue the situation in many cases, but not all.

Finally, the marriage or partnership may have been on the blink for some time and the woman has not been enjoying intercourse. The menopause is then used as a get-out clause, a reason to give up intimate relations. The majority of us women feel more in control of our lives when we are done with periods, premenstrual tension and the risk of pregnancy. We have more of a say about when we have sex and what we enjoy – or don't enjoy. Often it is only at this stage that a couple begin to communicate properly on this intimate, but important, subject. This is especially relevant when the approach of the menopause brings a bundle of changes. These can seriously damage your happiness if you are unable to discuss any difficulties with your partner.

The Process of Intercourse

- Desire, libido
- Lubrication of the vagina

- Arousal in response to the stimulus of touch
- Orgasm: the final release after a build-up of sensation – the peak of sexual pleasure

Regular intercourse should bring with it:

- The reassurance that you are sexually attractive
- Emotional satisfaction from your sexual behaviour

Many women, particularly those who are in the habit of having intercourse regularly, take the menopause in their stride, barely aware of any change and adjusting automatically – for instance by spending longer on foreplay. Others – about 50% – do run into difficulties and may even find intercourse painful: this is known as *dyspareunia*.

Problems Caused by a Reduction in Oestrogen

- Thinning and loss of elasticity of the lining of the vagina, making sexual activity uncomfortable. The delicate membrane may bleed.
- Lubrication of the vagina is slower to occur, and the volume of fluid is reduced: a dry vagina means painful intercourse.
- Urinary difficulties, including infection and poor control

What to Do

One obvious answer is to take HRT or, if you have had a hysterectomy, an oestrogen-only preparation. There may be medical reasons for you to avoid HRT, however. You may be a smoker, experience unpleasant side-effects or perhaps have been on the medication for several years and feel it wise to stop. You may manage satisfactorily with lubricants like KY jelly, an acetic acid moisturizer, or one of the alternative vaginal creams, Comfrey or Calendula, which also relieve itching and burning. Motherwort, Aloe Vera or Evening Primrose Oil by mouth are alternative recommendations.

Keeping in Practice
This is the greatest help of all, and absolutely essential. Intercourse itself stimulates the lubricating glands better than any other treatment – and there is also a psychological and emotional spin-off. You need to have intercourse a minimum of three to four times a month to keep the vaginal lining healthy and flexible and this also wards off the risk of urinary problems. As with other assets – if you don't use it, you lose it.

Lubrication
The natural supply may be enough in some women, but falls off in the older age groups:

- Age 50-60: 48% have adequate natural lubrication
- 60-70: 35% have adequate natural lubrication
- 70s: 23% have adequate natural lubrication

Sexual Self-soothing
If you are in the situation of having no available partner, either temporarily or longer term, do not despise masturbation. It is an ugly-sounding word with overtones of Victorian prudery, but it is a safe, dignified answer to a common problem. Approximately fifty per cent of women over 50 live alone for one reason or another, while over-70s of either sex are often without a partner. If it is your way of having sex, make it special – warm and comfortable with music playing and the telephone off the hook. It will evoke memories of happy physical experiences from the past and keep them alive – and it is as effective a physiological stimulus as intercourse for lubrication and achieving orgasm.

What Other People Do
Those having intercourse at least once a week:
- 50s: 73% – of these, 50% say they use different positions
- 60s: 63%
- 70s: 50%

From about age 68, most men cannot rely on having and keeping an erection, and full intercourse tails off. That leaves plenty of affectionate physical activity to enjoy.
- 80s, 90s, indefinitely: 90% of us enjoy kissing, cuddling and bodily closeness.

Those using self-soothing, always or sometimes:
- 50s: 47%
- 60s: 37%
- 70s: 27%
- 80s and 90s: 23%

Orgasm
At 50-plus, most women say they reach orgasm 50% of the time with sexual intercourse, but more often with masturbation. It depends partly on testosterone, but much more on psychological factors – like libido.

Libido, Sexual Drive – and Orgasm
The feeling that you want to have some sexual activity may continue at any age, but it can also switch off like a light at the menopause. Arousal – the erotic response to stroking and touching the trigger areas –may also go into abeyance. This change is not due to lack of oestrogen so much as the

simultaneous reduction in testosterone, the male hormone. The ovaries also produce this, in small quantities, before the menopause, and the supply is reduced in line with oestrogen. It is this hormone that is responsible for sexual interest in general, desire, drive and arousal, the response to a sexual stimulus. Again, the symptom of lost libido is most severe in the case of a surgical menopause when there is a sudden complete cut-off of the supply of testosterone.

Aphrodisiacs – sexual stimulants – have been used by men in particular, but women also, for hundreds of years. Commonly used are honey, chocolate and cocoa (Charles II's favourite), ginseng, ginger and yohimbine. Cannabis and alcohol are often used today in the hope of improving the sexual experience, but their effect is relaxation but a lessening of sexual drive. Sildenafil (Viagra) undoubtedly helps impotent men, but in women its only positive effect is an increase in the blood flow to the genital area.

A small dose of testosterone (5 mg daily of methyltestosterone by mouth, or the implant of a pellet) has been tried in some cases, but giving male hormone to a woman may have unwanted effects. These include an increase in body hair but a loss of head hair, acne, increase of weight, increase in cholesterol and headaches – everything you do not want. It is safer to stick to herbal remedies. The one with the best reputation as an aphrodisiac, and for relieving vaginal dryness and leading to wonderful orgasms, is a decoction (liquid extract) of Muira-Puama, plus Ginkgo Biloba.

Feeling sexy, all the way to orgasm, depends on several factors – emotional as well as hormonal. A plus for our sex is that we continue to be capable of orgasm, even multiple orgasm, into the most senior years, when men can only think and talk about it.

Hysterectomy

This operation affects 20% of women past the menopause. It can be a big stumbling block to the enjoyment of intimate relations around the change and later. Although there is no physical need for the presence of the uterus, anxiety occurs fairly frequently after a hysterectomy. It can cause headaches, restlessness, dry mouth and sometimes chest pain, as well as a sense of panic. This is far from conducive to a warm, happy relationship, and calls for gently supportive counselling.

Case Studies
Helena was 44 when she had her hysterectomy. She had been having extremely heavy periods due to a cluster of fibroids. Since she was under 45 and her ovaries were healthy, there was no necessity to remove them at

the same time. Helena did not want to experience the sudden development of severe menopausal symptoms that often follows removal of the ovaries (oophorectomy). She had recently remarried and her new husband already had two grown-up sons, so it suited her to have no worry about pregnancy. On the other hand, she very much wanted a generous, rewarding sex life.

Helena's doctor reassured her that there was no physical or hormonal reason for her sex life to be impaired, and quoted the crude saying that the operation meant that she had lost the nursery but still had the playpen. He did admit, however, that having a hysterectomy often brings on the menopause up to two years sooner than average. In fact Helena's change came on gently, when she was 49, and she went straight onto HRT. This kept her hormonal status near normal and she noticed no alteration in her sexual feelings. She was pleased that it also gave her some protection against osteoporosis and heart disease, and helped to maintain the youthful condition of her skin, hair and nails.

Enid's hysterectomy, when she was 60, included the removal of both ovaries and the cervix. She had developed a cancer of the endometrium (womb lining) and this was a safety measure. Enid was anxious and depressed and felt she had lost her femininity with her womb. In practical terms, as she had already passed the menopause and her ovaries had retired from egg and hormone production, she'd lost nothing by having them removed. She needed treatment, with chats to boost her confidence and a small dose of a relaxing antidepressant. Her doctor chose lofepramine (Gamanil), one 70-mg tablet daily. She feels she could enjoy sex again in the future, but doesn't feel quite ready yet.

Other Influences that Can Affect Your Sex Life

- You may never have had a particularly rampant sexual drive, but have been too busy to worry about it until now.
- Sex may feel no more exciting than cleaning your teeth, with the same old partner for so long.
- You may have developed your appetite for food and drink in recent years, so that your sexual appetite takes second place.
- A mix of embarrassment and fear of failure – you know that your children are faintly shocked that you can contemplate a sexual relationship – at your age!
- You feel unattractive. You may have put on weight and feel that you've lost your figure; your hair may be far from luxuriant and have gone grey; your skin shows wrinkles and your chin sags – but look around you: Is your partner as good as new? Or has he a pot belly and no hair to speak of?

Depression

This kills sexual and any other interest, and can creep up on you unrecognized in middle age, or as a response to the menopause.

The symptoms of a depressive illness are a low mood, with feelings of worthlessness, hopelessness or guilt, insomnia (including waking in the small hours), loss of appetite (often with weight loss), lack of energy and an inability to concentrate. HRT works miracles for some women in these circumstances, restoring self-confidence and a sense of well-being, but others respond better to antidepressant treatment – and if you are keen to avoid pharmaceuticals, St John's Wort is one good alternative.

This is also the time to give yourself a tonic by an overhaul of your appearance – skin, teeth, hair, shape and clothes. Give yourself the glow of good health with sensible amounts of food, sleep, exercise, fresh air and FUN. Never think it does not matter how you look, and even if you have health problems you can achieve the appealing charm of well-cared-for delicacy.

Your Skin

Use bath oils, never soaps or detergent-based bubble baths; use a moisturizer on your face and hands; do not let the sun shine directly on your face; cut out – or down on – booze and tobacco; finally, cultivate people who make you smile – a cross, anxious or glum expression and the lines that go with it are supremely unattractive.

Teeth

Make a friend of your dentist – he or she can make your smile a delight or a give-away. Have you any chipped or discoloured teeth that would benefit from capping? If you have dentures that are inclined to shift when you laugh or bite into something, particularly the lower ones, give your confidence a tonic with a new set – they will last for years.

Hair

It is more delicate than when you were in your 20s and 30s, and needs treating kindly – do not drag a comb through it when it is wet or douse it in harsh chemicals. Use the simplest shampoos, but often, and moisturizing conditioners; choose a short style unless your hair is thick enough to sweep up and give your facial contours a lift. Beware of hair dyes – a dark one can make you look like a witch and a blonde one makes your skin look muddy by comparison.

Make-up

The trick is to use all the help you can get, but in an under-stated way – a light, warm shade of foundation, dusted with translucent powder; eye, eyebrow and lip preparations used so lightly that no one realizes they are there. In particular, avoid bold lines, strong colours and glossy lipstick.

Clothes
These catch the eye sooner than your face and hair. It is unwise to go for bright, garish colours, but far worse to plump for 'safe' dull beige, mauve, fawn or grey or most little floral prints. Rust, sage, bluebell or deep rose may serve, and navy is kinder than black. Warning: Check how your skirt falls when you are getting out of a low chair or car seat – it's only OK for teens and twenties to reveal a flash of thigh. Jeans and trousers are fine – but not if your weight has become concentrated in your hips and bottom.

How you stand and walk make or mar the overall impression. Remind yourself not to stoop, slouch or waddle but to be as upright as possible. Finally, if you have put on a few surplus pounds, review your diet. Exercise tones you up, but you can only correct your weight if you also cut down on fats and sugary foods.

You may not be mistaken for a Hollywood starlet, but you need to believe in yourself – you are an intelligent, friendly, charming and attractive woman, who deserves the best in life.

Chapter 17

Contraception

There has been a revolution in the age when women start their families. It is no surprise, nowadays, to hear of someone having a baby in her late 40s or beyond, even a first-timer. Cheri Blair provided a particularly happy example of a successful pregnancy in the mid-40s.

Nevertheless, there are disadvantages:

- The risk of miscarriage from age 40 increases to 25-0%, compared with 10-15% in younger women. In older women, 40% of pregnancies do not run to term, for one reason or another.
- There is an increased risk of the baby having Down's syndrome:
  At 20 the risk is 1 in 2,000
  At 30 it is 1 in 350
  At 40 it is 1 in 100
  − but there is no increase in malformations with age.
- Diabetes and high blood pressure are more likely during pregnancy in older mothers, as − more dangerously − are haemorrhage or embolism
- Babies tend to have a low birth weight, and stillbirth is more frequent, although still rare.
- Fibroids can get in the way of the placenta or impede the birth itself.
- Most mothers of 40-plus require a Caesarean section.

In the future, when people are all living to 110, we may have ovary transplants and become fertile again in our 70s − but for the present it is safer not to have babies when you are already in the perimenopause.

Since sex remains an abiding pleasure and the cornerstone of most intimate relationships, if you are heterosexual and sexually active you will need to continue with contraception into your 50s − unless you have had a hysterectomy. The rule of thumb is:

- Over 50: continue contraception until 12 months after your final period
- Under 50: continue until you are 53.

You may be starting or may have already started on hormone replacement therapy (HRT), but this is not a contraceptive − the dosage of oestrogen is too small.

113

Combined Oral Contraceptive Pill

Apart from the contraceptive aspect, there are other benefits from taking the most popular form of contraceptive, the COC or combined oral contraceptive pill, in the run-up to the menopause and afterwards:

- It ameliorates heavy or irregular bleeding
- It checks the growth of fibroids
- It improves resistance to benign (non-cancerous) breast disease
- It helps with symptoms of the premenstrual syndrome.

All these tend to become more troublesome as the menopause approaches.

In addition, the contraceptive pill provides some protection against cancers of the ovary and uterus.

How It Works

The 'combination' in the combined oral contraceptive comprises oestrogen and progestogen. Together they suppress the production, by the pituitary gland in the brain, of the two hormones FSH (follicle stimulating hormone) and LH (luteinizing hormone), which trigger the monthly release of an ovum or egg. This is ovulation. Other effects are thickening of the mucus in the neck of the womb so the sperm cannot easily get through, and a thinning of the womb lining so that an embryo cannot develop there.

There is a wide choice of contraceptive pills, but since most of the side-effects are down to the oestrogen, it is sensible to choose a low-dose preparation – that is, one with fewer than 50 micrograms (mcg) of oestrogen per tablet.

When NOT to Take the Pill

In some cases the Pill should NOT be taken, if you suffer from certain problems or conditions affecting various organs or systems of the body:

- *Heart and blood vessels*: If you have relatives who have had a thrombosis; diabetes with artery problems; moderately or severely raised blood pressure; high cholesterol level; heart disease affecting the valves or rhythm; sickle cell anaemia
- *Liver*: jaundice; any form of liver disease; hepatitis A, B or C; cirrhosis; gallstones
- *General*: cancer; lupus; Crohn's disease; obesity; fibroids; heavy smoking
- *Drugs which interact with the COC*: tetracycline, carbamazepine (Tegretol), phenytoin (Epanutin), primidone (Mysoline), phenylbutazone (Butacote).

Stop the Pill at once if you experience any of these symptoms:
- Acute vision or hearing upset
- Severe headache
- Jaundice

Also, if you have to have a major operation, you cannot take the Pill for six weeks before and as long as you are in bed afterwards.

Combined Oral Contraceptives
21-day Type
With these you start on Day 1 of your cycle, continue daily for 21 days, then stop for 7 days for a 'period' – really a withdrawal bleed from stopping the hormones

Loestrin 20	(20 mcg oestrogen)
Mercilon	(20 mcg oestrogen)
Femodette	(20 mcg oestrogen)
Loestrin 30	(30 mcg oestrogen)
Microgynon 30	(30 mcg oestrogen)
Ovranette	(30 mcg oestrogen)
Ovran 30	(30 mcg oestrogen)
Eugynon 30	(30 mcg oestrogen)
Minulet	(30 mcg oestrogen)
Marvelon	(30 mcg oestrogen)
Femodene	(30 mcg oestrogen)
Brevinor	(35 mcg oestrogen)
Norimin	(35 mcg oestrogen)
Cliest	(35 mcg oestrogen)
Ovysmen	(35 mcg oestrogen)
Ovran	(50 mcg oestrogen)
Norinyl-1	(50 mcg oestrogen)

Phasic Type
This method reduces the total amount of hormone you take, by adding the progestogen partway through the cycle. The pills must be taken in the right order, then you again have a 7-day gap without medication.
- BiNovum
- TriNovum
- Synphase
- Logynon
- Trinordiol
- Tri-Minulet
- Triadene

ED (Every Day) Combined Type

These come in packs containing 7 placebo (inactive) tablets in 28. Start on Day 1 of your cycle and work through the tablets in order, without a break – then straight onto the next pack.

- Logynon ED
- Microgynon ED
- Femodene ED

Progestogen-only Contraceptives

No one knows quite how they work, but these are safer than COCs if you have diabetes, high blood pressure, smoke or you are an older women. Start on Day 1 of a cycle and continue with 1 tablet daily without a break.

- Femulen
- Micronor
- Microval
- Neogest
- Norgeston
- Noriday

Do not take these if you have serious disease of the arteries (atheroma), or have jaundice now or have had it in the past.

Stop the tablets at once if you have any hint of clotting (calf pain), migraine-type headache or disturbance of your vision.

How to Take the Contraceptive Pill

Whichever type of pill, take it if possible at the same time every day, preferably a few hours before the usual time of intercourse. Regular timing is particularly important with the progestogen-only pill; if you miss your regular time by three hours or more, this counts as a missed day, and you must be careful about intercourse accordingly. For the combined types, a 12-hour delay counts as a missed day.

Depot Preparations

These types of contraception are usually administered by injection.

- Depo-provera: injection every 12 weeks
- Mirena: intrauterine progestogen device which lasts 5 years
- Implanon: implant under the skin, to last 3 years

Do not take any of these in circumstances which contraindicate other forms of progestogen, for instance if you have jaundice or atheroma.

Other Contraceptive Arrangements

- Intrauterine devices (IUCDs) – do not use if you are anaemic or have heavy periods
- Spermicides
- Diaphragms
- Condoms

None of these should be relied upon alone.

Emergency Contraception

Schering PC4: oestrogen/progestogen COC. Take 2 tablets as soon as possible after intercourse, but within 72 hours. Repeat the dose in 12 hours. If you vomit within two hours of taking either dose – repeat. Have a pregnancy check in three weeks.

Levonelle-2: levonorgestrel 750 mcg (progestogen-only). Take 1 tablet as soon as possible after intercourse, but within 72 hours. Repeat the dose in 12 hours – then as for Schering PC4.

Side-effects of Contraceptives

Contraceptives, especially the Pill, are frequently blamed for almost any symptom or problem that arises while they are being taken. Putting on weight is a common such complaint, but it is seldom due to the medication. In fact, as many women lose two or three pounds when they start taking the Pill as gain weight. Symptoms of the irritable bowel syndrome – bloating and discomfort in the abdomen and upset bowels – are often put down to a COC. Similarly with loss of sexual interest – this can be caused by a multitude of emotional situations, or almost any physical illness.

Nevertheless, some of us do suffer one or another side-effect from a contraceptive. Fortunately there is such a wealth of formulations available from the different pharmaceutical companies that there is a good chance that you will find one that suits you. At the worst you can employ a barrier (condom or diaphragm) plus a spermicide. The risk of pregnancy is still only 1 in 5,000 if you are meticulous in your use of this method.

Possible Side-effects of Oral Contraceptives containing oestrogen (usually COCs)
- Swelling of the breasts, discomfort
- Bloating of the abdomen
- Fluid retention

- Cramps and pains in the legs
- Headaches
- Nausea
- Weight gain
- Breakthrough bleeding – spotting
- Brown patches on face
- Vaginal discharge
- Depression
- Loss of libido (sexual interest)
- Increased risk of blood clots – leg veins (DVT), stroke
- Increased blood pressure
- May increase the risk of breast cancer

Possible Side-effects of Progestogen-only Preparations
- Cysts of the ovary
- Clotting – especially of deep calf veins
- Tender, uncomfortable breasts
- Irregular bleeding
- Acne
- Headaches

Possible Side-effects with Other Methods
IUCDs: persistent bleeding; pain and cramps; slow pulse; asthmatic attack; epileptic fit

Depot preparations: prolonged, heavy or irregular bleeding; headache; abdominal pain; fluid retention with swelling; dizziness; weight gain

Implants: headache; tender breasts; hair loss; weepiness; acne; period pain; depression

Spermicides: no side-effects except in cases of special sensitivity to the chemical or the perfume that goes with it.

Barrier methods have no side-effects.

Chapter 18

Eating for Health in the Change

Eating is a pleasure we can enjoy all our lives – refreshment to the spirit and a restorative to the body. It underpins our health and strength, and our defences against disease.

It is easy to take our nourishment for granted and choose what we eat by habit – but this is a key time for making a reappraisal of your body's nutritional needs.

It is easy to understand that an infant's requirements differ from those of a child running about, and that the revolutionary bodily changes of puberty and motherhood call for equally dramatic modifications in the diet. While everybody knows that the menopause means change, most of us carry on eating just the same foods in just the same amounts as before. Yet our body's needs vary according to our changing lifestyle. It no longer has to prepare physically every month for the possibility of pregnancy, and life is no longer complicated by fitting in childcare with a job. It means we are free to follow new interests and undertake new activities – or perhaps those we could only dream of until now.

Physical Changes in the Perimenopause

- Lighter bones – with less manual-type work, they need not be so heavy
- Reduced muscle power, for the same reason, with about 35 kg of muscle compared with 40 kg earlier
- Slower metabolic rate, since you will not have the sudden severe demands of the reproductive years. At 45 it runs at 12%, compared with 25% previously
- The liver shrinks somewhat, since the metabolic needs are less – but this does mean you cannot detoxify alcohol as quickly as before
- Reduction in the size and function of the womb and ovaries

All of these changes are geared to economize on the amount of effort needed for maximum efficiency. The only change which is not helpful is an increase in the proportion of fat in the body, mainly within the abdomen.

Planning Your Eating

What you want your food to do for you:
● Supply you with energy
● Keep you warm
● Repair and replace worn or injured tissues
● Fight infection and other diseases through the immunity system

This is all powered by the slow combustion of fuel – your food.
Basic food groups – you need some of all three, since they work together:
● Proteins – essential for repair work
● Carbohydrates – for energy
● Fats – for stored energy. Fats have a bad press, but they are vital for the transportation and absorption of calcium and vitamin D. Two fatty acids, Omega-3 and Omega-6, reduce the amount of harmful LDL cholesterol, the type which causes heart disease and stroke, and increase the proportion of the 'good' HDL type.

Special Requirements

Care for Your Heart and Arteries
Before the approach of the menopause, women are protected by their hormones, mainly oestrogen, from the silting up of their arteries with fatty deposits – atheroma. This is the basic cause of coronary disease, high blood pressure and stroke. After the menopause we become as vulnerable to these nasties as men. The shortage of oestrogen can be countered to some extent by HRT, or more gently with phyto-oestrogens in the diet.

Sources of Phyto-oestrogens
● Soya and tofu are the richest suppliers, but soy sauce is too salty for a healthy diet
● Legumes: the pea and bean family, including chick peas, mung beans and lentils
● Other vegetables
● To take as food supplements: red clover, alfalfa, vervain

Omega-3 and -6 fatty acids also help to reduce the risk of atheroma. They are available in fish oils, particularly fatty fish such as salmon, sardines, mackerel and herring, and in cod-liver and halibut liver-oils. This is why nutritionists advise at least two fish meals per week. They can also be taken as supplements.

Care for Your Bones
Osteoporosis is the other big health danger of the menopause, and the main dietary need to combat it is calcium.

Sources of Calcium
Dairy products are the chief providers – you need the equivalent of a pint of milk a day – 672 mg – whether as liquid, yoghurt or cheese.

Milk, one-third of a pint:

	Full cream	*224 mg*
	Semi-skimmed	*231 mg*
	Skimmed	*235 mg*
	Longlife	*224 mg*

Yoghurt, small pot:

	Natural	*180 mg*
	Low fat, with fruit	*170 mg*

Dairy ice cream 100 g   *130 mg*

Cheese, 50 g/2 oz:

	Cheddar	*400 mg*
	Parmesan	*610 mg*
	Cottage	*60 mg*
	Edam	*370 mg*
	Danish blue	*290 mg*

Nuts and seeds, 100 g/3 1/2 oz:

	Almonds	*250 mg*
	Brazils	*180 mg*
	Walnuts	*60 mg*
	Fresh coconut	*13 mg*
	Sesame seeds	*670 mg*

Fish, 100 g/3 1/2 oz:

	Fried cod, haddock	*95 mg*
	Tuna, canned	*7 mg*
	Sardines, canned	*460 mg*
	Pilchard, canned	*168 mg*

Bread, 100 g/3 1/2 oz:

	Wholemeal	*23 mg*
	White	*100 mg*
	Malt	*94 mg*

Most plant foods contain very little calcium, or it is unavailable because of the presence of oxalates. The exception is dried figs.

Most meat – beef, lamb, poultry, ham – contains only tiny amounts.

What helps the absorption of calcium: Vitamin D, carbohydrates eaten at the same time, exercise.

What inhibits its absorption: phytates, found in husks of cereals especially oats and wheat; oxalates, found in rhubarb, spinach, strawberries and dandelion leaves; caffeine, especially filter coffee; phosphates as in fast foods, processed foods and cola drinks.

Alcohol, tobacco and salt also inhibit the proper use of calcium.

Care for Your Blood

Iron-deficiency anaemia is only too common at this stage in your life. It often creeps up unnoticed. The only early symptom is having less energy, but when it has become severe when you will be pale, have attacks of dizziness and even faint, and suffer palpitations and poor memory. You need iron.

Iron in Your Food

Best sources: liver, corned beef, fresh beef and lamb, oatmeal, old-fashioned treacle.

Next best: eggs, dark chocolate, peas, beans, Allbran, wholemeal bread.

Better than nothing: fish, milk, nuts, fruit, root vegetables.

Contrary to its reputation, spinach is next to useless as a supplier of iron, as you would need mammoth helpings to provide a noticeable amount. This goes for most green vegetables, for instance broccoli, cabbage and sprouts.

What helps its absorption: vitamin C, calcium in dairy food taken at the same time.

What hinders absorption: phytates in oats, wheat and all unmilled cereals; and tea – coffee is OK.

If you are prescribed iron for anaemia, DO NOT take the tablets with or after a meal. Iron is absorbed better taken BEFORE a meal. Space the doses out, since your body will not take in any more iron for up to six hours after the previous dose.

Folate and Vitamin B12 are also needed for making blood.

Folates are found in fresh green vegetables, especially spinach and broccoli, and in liver.

Vitamin B12 is found only in food from animal sources, and must be given by injection if you are a vegan. For everyone else, Vitamin B12 never runs short.

Care for Your Bowels

Constipation can be the bugbear of the menopausal age group, and irritable colon, diverticular disease and cancer of the colon are all more likely if your bowels are working sluggishly. This is a problem of our Western culture; it does not affect people in Asia and Africa. The big difference is the deficiency of fibre in our modern, over-refined, over-processed diet.

Fibre is not nourishing in the normal sense of the word, but it is essential to the healthy working of the bowel. It provides bulk, the necessary stimulus for the muscles of the colon, preventing harmful stagnation and uncomfortable constipation.

There are two types of fibre: soluble and insoluble. The soluble kind, in pectin, guar and oat fibre, causes a reduction in cholesterol. Oatmeal, oat bran, peas, beans and fruit all contain soluble fibre. Four portions of these daily provide 5 g of fibre – enough to lower the cholesterol concentration by 5%.

Wheat, wheat bran and other cereal fibre come in the insoluble group. Aim at a total fibre intake of 12 to 32 g (half to 1 oz) daily.

The Sources
● Bran, bran cereals such as Allbran
● Wholemeal, oatmeal, brown rice
● Dried fruit, especially prunes
● The jackets of jacket potatoes
● Fresh fruit, especially bananas
● Salads, green vegetables, nuts

Side-effects: You may produce an excess of gas in your bowel, causing pain and bloating.

Anti-ageing Foods
These are the antioxidants. Vitamin E is the principal one.
Sources
● Plant oils – wheatgerm, linseed, corn, peanut, coconut, and those found in the phyto-oestrogens soya beans, sunflower seeds, sesame seeds, beans
● Spreads with added vitamin E
● Cereal products
● Eggs
● Vitamins A and C
● Fresh, dark green vegetables

Foods that Suppress the Immune System
● Coffee, tea and such stimulants as Speed and cocaine
● Too much vitamin D
● Alcohol and cannabis
● Stress, pollution and lack of exercise and fresh air

Weight Control

This is a key time to pare off any unwanted pounds, because they become increasingly difficult to shift from the menopause onwards – especially below the waist.

General Guidelines for Reducing Weight
- Eat three meals a day, with drinks in between (elevenses, tea-time, late evening) and on waking
- No butter, spreads, cream, full-cream milk, fried foods
- No made-up meat dishes: burgers, sausages; pate, meat pies
- No chocolate, avocado, pastry, gateau
- No biscuits except crispbreads
- Moderate intake of alcohol and fruit juice (even unsweetened)

BUT you must have:

Carbohydrate: Three times daily: bread, toast, rolls, crispbread, potatoes, rice, bananas, porridge, bran cereal

Protein: Twice daily: fish, chicken, eggs, meat, cottage cheese, fromage frais, soya, yoghurt, baked beans

You may take freely: fresh fruit, salad, vegetables

High-fibre Diet

This has the added benefit of warding off constipation.

On Waking 2 cups of hot tea	*Tea-time* Tea, oatcakes or crispbread with honey
Breakfast Mineral water, juice, tea or coffee Porridge, bran cereal or muesli with stewed prunes Wholemeal toast, oatcake or crispbread with spread and chunky marmalade Coffee or tea (you may want to opt for herbal tea)	*Supper* Meat or equivalent (fish, cheese, beans) Jacket potato Salad or vegetables Fresh fruit or fruit pudding with dried or other fruit, or stewed fruit with yoghurt Drink with or after the meal
Lunch Vegetable soup Wholemeal sandwich with salad or celery, cheese Fruit Half a grapefruit or juice	*Bedtime* Digestive biscuit, camomile tea or milk drink

Avoid white bread, white rice, pasta, cakes and pastries.

To avoid the discomfort of bloating, try not to eat too many lentils, baked beans, natural bran, peas and beans.

General Purpose Diet – for the Menopause

Early Morning
Tea or coffee, rich tea biscuit

Breakfasts
Remember, NEVER skip breakfast.
1. Porridge, semi-skimmed milk and honey or stewed fruit. Apple. Tea/coffee
2. Grilled tomatoes, mushrooms or baked beans on toast. Tea/coffee/herbal tea
3. Yoghurt, fruit, toast with spread and preserve. Tea, etc.
4. Boiled or poached egg, toast, orange or banana

Elevenses
Coffee/tea/juice. Apple or semi-sweet biscuit

Lunches
1. Jacket potato with tuna or cottage cheese, salad garnish
2. Soup, roll, yoghurt and fruit.
3. Chicken, cheese or tofu, sardine, or egg wholemeal sandwich with salad
4. Cheese or ham, with a tomato or pineapple. Roll or crispbreads. Coffee, etc.

Tea
Drink (hot or cold)

Suppers
Starters (optional): crudites, melon, fruit juice, garlic mushrooms
First course 2 – 4 oz
(50 – 100 mg) meat, fish, cheese, egg or soya protein in one of these dishes:

1. Stir-fried chicken and vegetables
2. Vegetable curry and brown rice
3. Grilled fish and vegetables
4. Steak and onions, jacket potato

Second course

1. Baked apple with sultanas, ice-cream
2. Fresh fruit and blueberry muffin
3. Apricot upside-down cake
4. Stewed fruit and fromage frais

Coffee with semi-skimmed milk
Herb tea at bedtime, if you wish.

Useful Addresses

UK

British Menopause Society, 36 West Street, Marlow, Bucks SL7 2NB. Tel: 01628 890199. www.the-bms.org/

The Daisy Network, PO Box 392, High Wycombe, Bucks GP15 7SH

Women's Health Concern, PO Box 1629, London SW15 2ZL. Helpline: 020 8780 3007. Fax: 020 8780 3945.

The Amarant Trust, 11 – 13 Charterhouse Buildings, London EC1M 7AN. Tel: 020 7401 3855 and 01293 413000.

Women's Health, 52 Featherstone Street, London EC1Y 8RT. Helpline: 020 7251 6580 (Mon, Wed-Fri 11 am-5 pm) Email: health@women shealthlondon.org.uk

Women's Nutritional Advisory Service, PO Box 268, Lewes, East Sussex BN7 2QN. Tel: 01273 487366. Fax: 01273 487576. www.wnas.org.uk/

National Osteoporosis Society, PO Box 10, Radstock, Bath BA3 3YB. Tel: (general) 01761 471771, (medical) 01761 472721. www.nos.org.uk. Email: info@nos.org.uk

US

The National Women's Health Information Center, 8550 Arlington Blvd, Fairfax, VA 22031. Tel: 1-800-994-9662. www.4woman.gov/search/

American Menopause Foundation Inc., 350 Fifth Avenue, Suite 2822, New York, NY 10118. Tel: 212-714-2389. Fax: 212-714-1252. www.americanmenopause.org. email: menopause@americanmenopause.org

North American Menopause Society, PO Box 94527, Cleveland, OH 44101-4527. Tel: 440-442-7550. Fax: 440-442-2660. www.menopause.org

Australia

Women's Health Queensland Wide, Tel: (07) 3839 9988. Fax: (07) 3831 7214. Email: whcb@womhealth.org.au

Index

Acne.......................... 65, 72, 109, 118
Aerobics 80, 83
Agoraphobia 32
Alcohol 18, 21-26, 34-37, 59, 85,
93, 109, 119-124
Alzheimer's disease 53-55
Androgens 14, 21, 59
Angina 37, 49, 50, 82
Antidepressant......22, 31, 33, 54, 78, 92
94, 110, 111
Antioxidant 9, 37, 55, 76, 123
Appetite 30, 33, 38, 99, 110

Balance................. 4, 39, 40, 49, 58, 82
Bereavement 28, 29, 35, 75, 92
Bisphosphonates........................... 42
Bloating 23, 25, 63, 69, 72, 117,
123, 125
BMI, Body Mass Index................71, 81
Brown-Sequard, Dr C 51

Calcium.......... 9, 14, 22, 36, 40-43, 60,
104, 120-122
Callisthenics............................... 83
Cancer
- breast.... 42-46, 52-57, 60-64, 71-76,
101, 102, 118
- colon........................ 8, 52, 53, 82
- womb............................... 60, 74
Cereals................. 8, 48, 101, 122, 123
CHD, coronary
heart disease 6, 45, 59, 61
Cholesterol
- HDL 45-47, 64, 120
- LDL....................... 45, 46, 81, 120
Climacteric 6, 9
Clitoris 10
Constipation.. 8, 23, 33, 39, 86, 122-124
Contraceptive 16, 17, 32, 52, 55, 58,
60, 63, 72, 75, 113-117
Coffee........... 19, 21, 24, 26, 34, 37, 48,
64, 69, 70, 73, 83, 85, 122-125
Collagen.............................14, 21, 22
Colon - Irritable 72, 98
Cupping 26
Cystocoele 18

Depression.. 4, 29-34, 54, 72-82, 94, 97,
102, 104, 111, 118

DEXA, dual energy
X-ray absorptiometry.............. 41, 42
Diabetes 45, 47, 57, 71, 77-81, 85,
113-116
Disease
- cardiovascular 44-50, 53
- coronary heart 6-9, 45, 50, 59, 61
Doderlein's bacillus 18
'Dowager's hump' 39
DVT, deep vein
thrombosis 74, 77, 78, 92, 118
Endometriosis..........9, 13, 17, 56, 87, 91
Evening Primrose oil...26, 63, 69, 74, 93,
103, 107

'Feminine Forever' 52
Fibre............ 8, 23, 26, 86, 93, 123, 126
Fibrocystic disease 74
Fibroids 9, 13, 16, 57, 77, 90, 113, 114
Fish liver oil 9, 39, 60
Fracture
- Colles.................................... 41
- hip 40, 41, 53, 81
- shoulder 41
- vertebral 38, 40
- wrist 41
Fruit ...8, 9, 48, 76, 86, 101, 102, 121-125

Gallstones........................... 57, 78, 114
Gels.......................59, 66, 72, 73, 93
Genetics 36, 37
Glucosamine 22
Glucose................................. 45, 81

Headache 8, 23, 25, 57-63, 72,
74, 96-100, 104, 109, 118
Height - loss of 38
Hepatitis.............................. 56, 114
High Blood pressure 9, 44, 46, 49,
50, 57, 71, 77-81, 99, 113, 116, 120
Hormones
- anabolic................................ 42
- growth.......................... 21, 42, 51
Hot flushes.......... 24-28, 52, 53, 61-69,
76, 85-87, 94, 97, 102, 103
HRT, hormone
replacement therapy..5, 8, 17-26, 31, 32,
37-46, 52-78, 85, 90, 99,
105-107, 110-113
Hyperventilation 31

Hysterectomy ... 6, 40, 53, 57-62, 77-92, 107, 109-113

IHD, ischaemic heart disease 44
Implants 21, 59, 67, 68, 72, 118
Incontinence 18-22, 53
Insomnia . 7, 34, 54, 74, 78, 100, 103, 111
Irritability 4, 23, 31, 63

Kegel, Dr A 20
Kyphosis 39

Laxatives 39
Libido 32, 59, 108, 118

Mammogram 23, 55, 74
Marriage 4, 17, 33, 54, 106
Mood swings 63, 72-78, 87, 104

Naturopathy 95, 97

Obesity 57, 71, 77, 114
Oestrogen ... 6-23, 37, 44-77, 82-94, 101, 102, 107-109, 113-117, 120
Oophorectomy 6, 61, 110
Osteoarthritis 14, 22, 40
Osteoporosis 6-8, 14, 22, 36-39, 42-44, 53, 60-64, 73-82, 101, 110, 121
Overweight ... 8, 9, 15, 28, 37, 45-47, 54, 55, 71, 75, 78, 80, 81
Ovulation 13, 14, 51, 53, 114

Pain
- abdominal 19, 38, 78, 118
- back 23, 25, 38, 75, 100
Palpitations 24, 25, 31, 53, 56, 59, 64, 69, 85, 94, 100, 122
Patches 65, 66, 69, 72, 75, 118
Perimenopause 6, 7, 23, 25, 44, 48, 60, 81, 113, 119
Pessaries 20, 93
PMT, PMS, premenstrual tension, premenstrual syndrome .. 4, 16, 23, 63, 64, 92
Progesterone ... 13-16, 23, 42, 45, 51-53, 59-64, 68, 72-76, 102
Prolapse 16, 18, 90
Psychotherapy - cognitive 33

Purdah 5
Quain, Dr R 9

Rectocoele 18
Relaxation 26, 35, 47, 72, 82, 95, 109

Self-esteem 27, 28, 71, 78-82
SERMS, selective (o)estrogen receptor modulators 42, 64, 76
Smoking 8, 9, 37, 46, 48, 55, 59, 80, 85, 114
SSRIs, selective serotonin re-uptake inhibitors ... 33, 78
Steroids 37, 43
Stoop 38, 39, 98, 112
Stress 9, 15, 20, 26, 35, 38, 47-50, 53, 75, 87, 100, 123
Stress-busters 9
Stroke 9, 14, 44-50, 118, 120
Sugar ... 8, 26, 45-48, 63, 64, 81, 95, 112
Suppository 68
Sweats 24, 25, 34, 52, 53, 59-69, 85, 94, 97, 101, 103

Tamoxifen 42, 64, 76
TCER, trans-cervical endometrial resection 88-90
Testosterone 15, 59, 65, 68, 71, 72, 75, 108, 109
TIA, transient ischaemic attack 49
Tibolone 64, 65
Thyroxine 37, 49
Tranquillizers 37, 94

Ultrasound 42, 74, 77
Underactive thyroid 71

Vegetables 8, 9, 48, 76, 101, 120, 122-125
Vertebra (-ae) 36-42, 82, 97
Vitamins 37, 69, 76, 87, 96, 104, 123
Vulva 10

Walking 9, 27, 34, 39, 80, 82-84
Weight - gain 8, 9, 15

X-ray 42